How to Ride a Dragon

362.1969944900922 Toc

Tocher, M.
How to ride a dragon.

How to Ride

a Dragon

WOMEN WITH BREAST CANCER TELL THEIR STORIES

MICHELLE TOCHER

illustrations by
JULIE DUBUC
foreword by
ELEANOR NIELSEN

KEY PORTER BOOKS

National Library of Canada Cataloguing in Publication Data

Tocher, Michelle
    How to ride a dragon : women with breast cancer tell their stories

Includes bibliographical references.

ISBN 1-55263-397-7

    1. Breast – Cancer – Patients – Biography.   2. Breast – Cancer – Psychological aspects.
I. Title. II. Series.

RC2806.B8T6195 2001   362.1'9699449'00922   C2001-902694-3

The publisher gratefully acknowledges the support of the Canada Council for the Arts
and the Ontario Arts Council for its publishing program.

We acknowledge the financial support of the Government of Canada through the Book
Publishing Industry Development Program (BPIDP) for our publishing activities.

Key Porter Books Limited
70 The Esplanade
Toronto, Ontario
Canada   M5E 1R2

www.keyporter.com

Design by Counterpunch/Linda Gustafson

Lyrics from *Puff the Magic Dragon* reprinted by permission of Warner Bros. Publications
and Cherry Lane Music Publishing

Printed and bound in Canada

01 02 03 04 05 06   6 5 4 3 2 1

Foreword

In 1996, a sports medicine research team at UBC, headed by Dr. Don McKenzie, recruited a small group of women with breast cancer to challenge the common wisdom of the day, which advised restrictions in strenuous upper body exercise for women after surgery and radiotherapy for breast cancer. The research involved training and monitoring the women as they learned the ancient sport of dragon boat paddling. Little did the research team know the excitement their study would generate. Five years later, breast cancer survivor dragon boat teams exist in over 30 communities from Victoria to Halifax.

How to Ride a Dragon is the culmination of a dream that began as I listened to women's stories and was moved by the beauty of so many tales of "everyday" heroism. These stories, combined with the enthusiastic support all teams receive at annual Dragon Boat Race Festivals, got me thinking about the absence of role models to help us overcome adversity in our lives.

One day I received a message from a paddler from another team that was headed "Truly an inspiration!!" It went on to say, "Every time your team came paddling down the race course, my paddling partners and I stood and applauded with hundreds of others watching along the course. It was fascinating watching people's reactions – you were all truly an inspiration. I think you sent everyone home that night a better person. The breast cancer challenge was the highlight of the weekend for me – I shed a tear or two and remembered family members who have died from breast cancer and other types of cancer. My only wish is that we all strive to be as gutsy and courageous as you all are. A job well done!"

Added to these thoughts was the knowledge that we, the survivor paddlers, are the lucky ones, and that there is much that needs to be done to conquer breast cancer, as there is much that needs to be done to conquer all cancers. Dragons Abreast, the Toronto team, was supportive of embarking on a book project and agreed to help to raise money for the Canadian Breast Cancer Research Initiative.

With all of this rolling around in my head, I had the good fortune to run into Michelle Tocher, a writer and story-teller whom I had worked with a few years back. It turned out that Michelle was also a lover of dragons and mythology and she leapt at the project. She proposed a mythological approach to the book which will unfold in the pages to follow. We hope you find solace in these tales and that all your dragons become companions on your journey through life.

Eleanor Nielsen

Acknowledgements

We are grateful to all the women who contributed to the creation of this book, especially to the 22 survivors across Canada who had the courage and the candor to share their stories. The book would not have been possible without them, nor without Eleanor Nielsen, who had the original vision to tell the story of breast cancer survivors who are dragon boating. We would also like to thank the members of the advisory group who oversaw the book's development, Akky Mansikka of Dragons Abreast, and Jane Frost of Abreast in a Boat; and all the survivors who reviewed the book, Chantal Brunet, Marian Busch, Bernice Kwasnicki, Marianne Primeau, Cathy Prusak, Anita Ewart, Marjorie Greenwood, Irene Hogendoorn, Julie Dubuc and Brenda Welsh. Thanks also to Jean Shepperd and Nan Brien for help with the final edit.

This was a project that had many supporters and two major patrons, Maritime Life and Scotiabank.

Maritime Life was the first to support our vision, making it possible to create this book. It was the culmination of three years of support for survivor dragon boating, including Toronto's Dragons Abreast for its first three years and Bosom Buddies of Nova Scotia for one year.

Scotiabank is a generous sponsor of breast cancer survivors teams. The organization first sponsored the original Vancouver team, Abreast in a Boat in 1997 and has since provided support to two additional teams: Toronto's Dragons Abreast and the North Bay Warriors of Hope.

Finally, thanks to Clare McKeon at Key Porter for being a fount of enthusiasm, and to Anna Porter for her love of dragons.

Eleanor Nielsen
Michelle Tocher

Scotiabank first sponsored the original Vancouver Abreast in a Boat team in 1997. Since then, this team has grown to over 100 women, all breast cancer survivors. These woman have inspired Scotiabank to provide support for two additional Dragon Boat teams: the Toronto Dragons Abreast and the North Bay Warriors of Hope. I hope that you enjoy *How to Ride a Dragon* and discover your own dragon-slaying within.

Peter C. Godsoe
Chairman and Chief executive Officer
Scotiabank

The Canadian Breast Cancer Research Initiative

Breast cancer is the most common cancer amongst women in Canada, accounting for about 20,000 new cases each year, over 5,000 deaths and the loss of about 95,000 years of potential life. An estimated 85,000 to 100,000 Canadian woman are living with breast cancer.

The proceeds of this book will be donated to the Canadian Breast Cancer Research Initiative through two of its funding partners, the Canadian Breast Cancer Foundation and the Canadian Cancer Society. Any further donations or inquiries can be directed to:

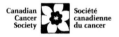

Canadian Breast Cancer Foundation, National Office
790 Bay St., Suite 1000
Toronto, ON
M5G 1N8

Canadian Cancer Society
10 Alcorn Ave., Suite 200
Toronto, ON
M4V 3B1

On behalf of all women with breast cancer, we thank you for your support.

Table of Contents

The dragon is the spirit of change... therefore of life itself... taking new forms according to its surroundings, yet never seen in its final shape. It is the great mystery itself. Hidden in the caverns of inaccessible mountains, or coiled in the unfathomed depth of the sea, he awaits the time when he slowly arouses himself into activity. He unfolds himself in the storm-cloud, he washes his mane in the darkness of the seething whirlpools. His claws are the fork of the lightning.... His voice is heard in the hurricane.... The dragon reveals himself only to vanish.

– Kakasu Okakura, *The Awakening of Japan*

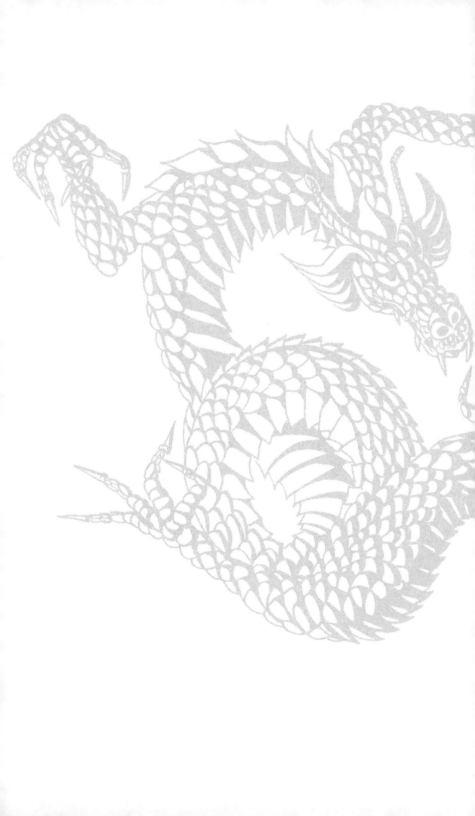

CHILD

Are all the dragons fled?
Are all the goblins dead?
Am I quite safe in bed?

NURSE

Thou art quite safe in bed
Dragons and goblins all are dead.

CHILD

When Michael's angels fought
The dragon, was it caught?
Did it jump and roar?
(Oh, nurse, don't shut the door.)
And did it try to bite?
(Nurse don't blow out the light.)

NURSE

Hush, thou knowest what I said,
Saints and dragons all are dead.

FATHER

(to himself)
Oh child, nurse lies to thee,
For dragons thou shalt see,
Please God that on that day
Thou may'st a dragon slay.
And if thou do'st not faint
God shall not want a Saint.

– H.D.C. Pepler, 1916

Introduction

When I first read Pepler's poem, I sided with the father. He wanted to prepare his child to meet the dragons of life, not lie and pretend they all were dead. I'm not sure that dragons *are* dead. They are certainly alive and well in myth and in our imaginations. If we have been challenged by a supreme fear, loss or illness, or forced to rally from the deepest place in our spirit, then surely we know what it means to meet a dragon.

Dragons have traveled with us since the beginning of time, and they are universal to the human experience. They appear in the folklore of nearly every culture around the world. Some authors argue that dragons are memories of those predators that we feared early on in our evolution. In *An Instinct for Dragons*, author David E. Jones writes that the dragon symbolized our ancestors' most feared enemies – those who attacked from the sky and from the ground. The dragon is a complex symbol which preserves within it our ancient fear of raptors, cats and snakes. It would be an easy theory to accept were it not for the fact that in many cultures of the world, especially Asian cultures, the dragon is benevolent. The dragon is the embodiment of wisdom and beneficence; as the bringer of rain and fertility, it is a magnificent and life-bestowing creature. So somehow the dragon has managed to acquire a contradictory nature – both ruthless destroyer and loving creator.

Being a teller of stories and myths, I have always been fascinated by dragons, but I haven't really understood what they symbolize. Under the surface of my consciousness there does seem to be a very real, instinctive knowledge of what it means to meet a dragon, and yet I confess that I don't seem to be able to get underneath, to understand what I know. Then, around the time I was beginning to wonder about the dragon, my father was diagnosed with esophageal cancer and his life was thrown into jeopardy. All of a sudden, his business ventures and traveling plans were swept aside and there was nothing before him but the threat of death. In my mind's eye, I kept seeing the dragon and my father marshaling all of his forces to meet it. I didn't know where the ordeal would take him or whether he would survive his deadly encounter but, like the child in the poem, I wanted to know so I would understand what he was going through and be better prepared to meet dragons of my own.

So began my search for dragon stories. I went looking for real live stories from people who could honestly say that they had met a dragon and survived. I also began reading mythological stories about dragons from cultures around the world. Then one day I was speaking on the phone with my friend Eleanor Nielsen, who worked at the Canadian Cancer Society. She told me that she had been nurturing a dream to develop a book about "dragon boaters" and my ears pricked up. In the mid '90s, Eleanor had started the first dragon boating team in Toronto for survivors of breast cancer, and she wanted to tell the powerful stories of the women. I knew nothing about dragon boating, so Eleanor gave me a little education. She explained that dragon boat racing was a sport which has been imported from China and goes all the way back to ancient times. A dragon boat has a dragon head and tail, and it carries 22 people, including a drummer who sits up front to keep the paddlers in time and a steersperson who stands in the back. Those who race dragon boats meet at festivals every summer to "ride the dragon," and the sport has drawn thousands of enthusiasts from corporations and organizations around the world.

There is a curious legend associated with dragon boating. During China's Warring State period (481–221 BC), there lived a poet named Qu Yuan, who was a trusted advisor to the King of Chu. Qu Yuan gave the King a piece of advice that he didn't appreciate and the King turned on the poet, banishing him to a remote area of southern China. Qu Yuan wandered the countryside, torn from his roots and filled with despair. When he learned that his beloved region of Chu had fallen to its rivals, he was shattered. And so on the fifth day of the fifth month, Qu Yuan clasped a huge rock to his breast and threw himself into the torrents of the Miluo River. News of his suicide spread through the countryside, and hundreds of local fishermen raced out in their boats in an attempt to save the poet. They beat their drums and splashed their paddles on the water to ward off the water dragons and keep them from eating his body. They scattered rice on the water to ensure that he would never grow hungry, and every year after they went out on the water in their dragon boats, re-enacting their attempt to save the poet and to keep the water dragons at bay.

Drawn to the Shore

After reading about dragon boating, I went to see a race that was taking place at a Toronto harbor. I stood with thousands of people gathered on the shore and watched the racers surge past. The boats seemed almost to fly off the surface of the water, especially those that were powered by paddlers with gleaming muscles and seriously trained bodies.

Then I began to sense a rousing excitement around me. People were jostling for space at the shoreline. Women in pink hats and shirts paddled six boats to the starting line, and I noticed that some of the people who had appeared along the shore were bearing pink carnations, including the woman who stood beside me. She had short gray hair, a rather colorless complexion and warm, friendly eyes. "What's going on?" I asked her.

"The breast cancer race is coming up," she replied. She gave me a warm smile.

"Oh, I've heard about this," I said. "Are you part of the team?"

"Yes," she said. "Only I'm not able to race any more."

I saw that she was pale and thin; she looked too fragile to be standing in the wind that blew hard off the water.

"What's the flower for?" I whispered.

"Watch and I'll show you," she said.

Six boats were lined up at the starting line – a colorful, happy crowd of ladies in pink – and even at a distance I could see they were not like the other racers. Women of every age, shape and size occupied those boats – paddling was not going to be easy for them. I looked around and noted the expressions of love and concern on the faces of the people around me. The starting gun went off and the boats leaped forward, the women paddling with all their might, plowing through the water to the beat of drums while the onlookers shouted encouragement. I couldn't see individual faces, but I could feel their struggle – it gripped my heart. You could see that they were fighting hard, that they were attacking the water with the ferocity of those who have fought the dragon and aren't finished fighting. When they crossed the finish line, one boat soared in ahead of the rest, and the crowd cheered wildly. After it had crossed the finish line, the winning boat turned while the other boats crossed over and the last labored in. The crowd cheered and whooped and hollered for the last boat just as it had for the first. Then the boatloads of women in pink did an unexpected thing.

They joined all their boats together.

Wave after wave of emotion rolled through me, through the crowd.

"This is how we remember those who are too sick to paddle, and those who have died," said the woman beside me, raising her flower into the air. The dragon boaters – all 146 women – raised their pink carnations, and in one motion they tossed their flowers onto the water, in unison with the people who bore flowers on the shore.

For a moment the crowd fell silent and then the women paddled in. I raced to the pier to see them disembark. A crowd of people had gathered, including all the other young, fit dragon boaters, and they were all applauding. I kept wondering, *What is going on here? Where is all this emotion coming from?* I thought of Qu Yuan and how he had flung himself into the river in despair. These women were doing more than dragon boat racing. They were doing more than winning races or even surviving breast cancer. They were surviving despair – celebrating in the face of death, living with the dragon of cancer.

The women in pink raised their paddles and formed a long archway to receive their teammates and competitors. I stood at the end of the corridor and watched them emerge one by one – exhausted, laughing, liberated, and dripping with water and tears.

There was no question in my mind that I had found the people who could tell me real, living stories about what it meant to meet and conquer dragons. So, with the generous support of Maritime Life, I began to develop a book that would fulfill Eleanor's dream to tell the survivors' stories. We decided to create a kind of "spirit boat" in the form of a book that would contain 22 stories of women from across Canada. We began by sending out a call to dragon boating survivors of breast cancer – to ask them what dragon boating meant to them and to determine if they were willing to tell their dragon stories. To our delight and amazement, 22 women came forward, including two steerspersons and a drummer, so we did indeed have a full "spirit boat"! (We have included profiles of all the women beginning on page 213.)

Over the year that followed, we sent a storytelling guide to our participants to draw out each of their experiences with breast cancer, dragon boating and the mythological dragon. In the storytelling guide and through our subsequent interviews, we asked them if they could mythologize their cancer as a dragon and, if so, tell us what it looked like, where it lived and how it appeared and struck. It was interesting that about two-thirds of the survivors were readily able to mythologize their cancer as a dragon and see themselves in the role of the dragon slayer. But the rest of them said that their dragon was not deadly; it was benevolent and was associated with the new opportunities that emerged in the aftermath of their cancer. Many of the women who associated their cancer with a dragon found that, in their engagement with the disease, the deadly creature transformed into a life-giving, providential companion.

So as I listened to the stories of the women and read books about dragons and dragon boating, a picture of the universal dragon began to emerge. I found that the Old English story of *Beowulf* reflected many of the living experiences that the women recounted in their struggle to slay the dragon of breast cancer. The author is not known, but the poem was probably written sometime in the 8th century AD, and although it was composed for an Anglo-Saxon audience who loved to hear heroic tales of the early North Germanic people, it continues to be relevant today. Nowhere in literature do we find such a vivid portrait of the deadly dragon and of the tasks of the dragon slayer.

But the dragon is not just a beast to be slain – myth and living experience suggest that there comes a time in our battle with dragons when war gives way to peace and acceptance, and out of that encounter a new kind of being emerges. Dragon and dragon slayer are transformed.

This is the story of those who have gone the whole distance with the dragon – who have been both dragon slayers and dragon lovers. It is the story I wanted to know above all when my father was diagnosed with a lethal form of cancer. It is the kind of story that prepares us and our children for the mortal challenges of life, showing us how to survive the unsurvivable, how to live fully in the shadow of death. The story of the "women in pink" performs the timeless task of dragon stories around the world – it prepares us to face the dragon that will inevitably meet us all.

How to Ride a Dragon

I

Dragon Strike

The story of Beowulf *begins when the Danish King Hrothgar decrees that a mighty feasting Hall be built where he can celebrate his victories and distribute his wealth. The towering Hall goes up and it is a wonder to behold. Wrought with gold, it glitters in the sun and is soon filled with happy revelers. Their laughter can be heard far and wide, along with the clear, ringing voice of the poet who endlessly sings the praises of the Almighty and of His perfect creations.*

Down in the gloom of the marshes and fens, a dragon named Grendel is disturbed by the noise from the Hall. Condemned by God to live in exile for the sins of Cain, Grendel prowls the moors, snarling with envy and rage. But the people do not hear the dragon's rumblings. Secure in the King's stronghold, they laugh and feast in their world of light.

THE UNDERWORLD DRAGON

Most of the women led fairly normal and secure lives before they were diagnosed with breast cancer. Some had been through stressful times but, like the King, they had secured order in their households. They were busy with families, work, and plans for the future, and few had any inkling that a disease might be rumbling within their "kingdoms."

When we asked them if they could mythologize their cancer as a dragon, more than half of the survivors had no trouble seeing their cancer as a cold, ruthless monster that suddenly burst upon the scene and engaged them in a desperate battle for life. Marianne Primeau of Winnipeg described her cancer as a dormant dragon that one day erupted out of nowhere and shattered everything.

> Mine was an inactive dragon that suddenly went crazy. I couldn't get a good look at it because, when it attacked, it turned my whole world upside down. First it was minding its own business in its own little world and all of a sudden it greeted me, and I thought, *Why did you pick on me, what do you want from me?*

Some women saw their dragons as huge monsters who terrorized the vicinity and left a path of destruction in their wake. Brenda Welsh of Toronto said that her cancer was like a dragon who came crashing through town and into her home.

> It lived in a faraway place and took a great deal of time to reach my doorstep. Along the way it killed entire villages of women. By the time it reached me, it was starting to tire. It was only by luck that it had weakened when it came to my home. It was large but agile and moved about undetected until it was ready to strike. It was sneaky and lurked around my home for several days, like a robber stakes out a house before it breaks in. Because of its sheer size it was able to cause chaos with little effort.

Some women felt that their dragons had been lying in wait for some time, observing their situation. Karen Kellner of Toronto saw her dragon as a lurking witness, waiting to strike: a terrible but strangely intimate associate.

🍃 Where did my dragon first reside? That's a good question. It wasn't in a deep dark cave hiding like a secret. It didn't live in the forest like a medieval dragon would. I think it lived close to my house, up above in a high tree or in the clouds where it could see me... and when I had reached the end of my tether, it paid me a visit.

Other dragons slept and woke deep within the earth. Franci Finkelstein of Toronto felt that her dragon lived underground and awoke when the weather warmed.

🍃 My dragon was definitely a fire breather. Its skin was green as an avocado, with a texture soft as lamb's leather. It had scales and small wings by its side, but it had a wingspan of 20 feet. My dragon appeared timid when it was resting peacefully, and it had a certain warmth. It lived in a dark, cool cavern with only one light piercing in through a small hole the size of a manhole, way up at the earth's surface, 30 feet above.

In the cave there was a secret passage that the dragon could skillfully slide through when it entered my world – "the real world." It rested for a long while, and then, as summer drew near and the days warmed and lengthened, the time came for that green-winged fire breather to slither out and find its prey!

The ways in which the survivors portrayed their dragons reflected the ways in which they experienced the destructive power of cancer. Their imagery often captured what they felt deeply but couldn't express in any other way. Franci imagined her dragon sleeping underground because it had already made its presence known in her family. Two years before Franci was diagnosed, her mother had breast cancer. Then her younger cousin Susie was diagnosed with a particularly aggressive form of colon cancer, which ended up taking her life. Franci, who was only in her mid-30s at the time of her cousin's illness, became alarmed by the presence of cancer in her family, and she felt that in some way it lay dormant inside her own being.

🌿 When my mother was diagnosed with breast cancer, my family was shocked. My mother's parents had gone through cancer, but when it happened to my own mother, I thought, *It's getting scary now.* Then when my cousin Susie was diagnosed, we all got scared.

Impelled by an inner warning, Franci asked for a mammogram when she went for a physical that winter.

🌿 I asked my doctor, "Should I have a mammogram?"
He said, "No, you're too young."
I thought, *No, don't say I'm too young.* There was something buried deep inside of me thinking, *It's going to be* me *next.*

The Dragon Strikes

Under the cover of night, Grendel creeps into the King's Hall where the warriors are soundly sleeping. Their bellies are full of wine and food, and their minds are dead to the sorrows of the world. Then, in a sudden and ravenous frenzy, the dragon seizes 30 men, butchers them and hauls their bodies off to his lair. At dawn the tragedy is discovered, and a wail goes up from the Hall. The King and his men rush to the scene. Stunned by the carnage, they retrace the dragon's bloody footprints that lead off into the gloomy fen.

Many survivors experienced their cancer as a dragon who attacked invisibly and secretively. The deadly nature of the creature was hard to fathom because on the surface there were no signs of ill health. Cancer stole in like Grendel, an "invisible enemy" who attacked in the dark, from within.

Marian Busch was working as a business systems consultant in Calgary when her cancer appeared. It was the summer of 1997 and she was 36 years old. Marian recalled that her work life had been extremely busy when she found the lump in her breast. She went to see her doctor and she booked an appointment for a biopsy. Nobody was overly concerned since she had a history of benign fibroadenomas (common, hard, non malignant lumps). When she went for her biopsy, Marian left her daily round of concerns and entered a subterranean realm.

> I found myself lying in the darkened room in the basement of the Grace Women's Health Centre, naked from the waist up, looking at the fuzzy pictures on the ultrasound screen – trying to see the lump in my right breast. After a few minutes, the radiologist and his intern came bustling into the room and we quickly covered off my previous medical history. Then he turned to the ultrasound and began complaining about how the lump was too small to do a needle biopsy.
>
> "I don't know why they bother me with these things," he said. "The needle is bigger than the lump."
>
> We discussed what to do as he completed a manual breast exam of my left breast. My breasts have always been quite dense and lumpy and so, once again, given my history [of having benign fibroadenomas], I was sent home feeling like a silly goose with the assurance that "It's probably nothing. Don't worry about it."

It was not easy for Marian to extricate herself from her demanding work schedule in order to go for the excisional biopsy. Neither she nor her colleagues in the active, daylight world comprehended the gravity of the problem or its implications for the future.

For the next four months, Marian buried herself in her work and for the most part forgot about the lump. However, she had been put on watch for signs of danger. She couldn't tell if the lump had changed; yet the fact that it was there gnawed at the back of her mind. At her next annual physical the doctor recommended an excisional biopsy so they could find out, once and for all, what the lump was. Marian was relieved because at this point she just wanted to draw the mysterious thing out into the light of day.

> At the time of my diagnosis I was a busy professional, totally focused on my career, with strong workaholic tendencies. To a large extent my work ruled my life, and there was little time for me to pursue other interests or to keep in touch with family and friends. I worked – a lot. And while I enjoyed my work and was good at it, I resented the fact that work seemed to intrude into my entire life.
>
> The day I was to go for my excisional biopsy, I was working on a project with very tight timelines. We had been working feverishly to prepare for some upcoming workshops and it was going to be nip-and-tuck as to whether we could get everything done in time. My biopsy was scheduled for 11:00 on a Thursday morning. (It amazes me that I remember these details without having to look them up.)
>
> I went to the office early to get some work done and update my "To Do" list. I was going through a review of what was left to do with my teammate when the project manager came into my office. She wanted me to attend a meeting to help sort out some issues with one of the other teams. I begged off, saying that I had to finish what I was doing and then go for my biopsy.
>
> She became so insistent that I finally had to tell her, "In 30 minutes I am leaving for a biopsy. I'm sorry, but I cannot attend this meeting right now. You'll have to go ahead

without me or reschedule it for tomorrow."

I replay this scene in my mind and it is so familiar. I have never been very good at saying no, especially if there is something I can do to help. As a result, work ends up taking over my life, and I resent it. When I was diagnosed, I was tired to my soul, feeling burned out and struggling to find some balance in my life.

I went for the biopsy at the Grace Women's Health Centre in Calgary on Thursday, July 30, 1998. My husband, Ken, picked me up from work and drove me to the hospital. I was somewhat concerned but, given my history, I tried to calm my fears, telling myself that it was just another fibroadenoma and that everything would be fine. At that point, I was more concerned about the biopsy procedure itself. They would be using a local anesthetic, which meant that I would be awake through the procedure. I have had a number of local surgeries and, while they are not painful, they gross me out completely. I was tense, nervous and full of dread at the thought of more local surgery. More importantly, I was embarrassed that I was so upset by "such a little thing."

Dr. MacColl was wonderful and completed the surgery quickly and skillfully. The nurse talked to me about inconsequential things to take my mind off what was happening. Then it was done and they took the sample out to the lab. I breathed a sigh of relief and thought to myself, *There, that's over and you're fine now.*

When Dr. MacColl came back into the operating room, he said that he had not gotten all of the lump. He would have to reopen the incision and do it again. Alarm bells began quietly ringing in my mind. Having worked so hard to psych myself up for this, I reacted angrily. I had summoned all my emotional reserves to get through the first procedure and now I had to go through this again and I had to do it right now. I felt like a runner who has poured her heart and soul into a race only to be told that it had been a false start. I would have to go back and re-run the race right now, before I had a chance to recover. I struggled to compose myself, and in a few minutes it was all over – again.

I got dressed and my husband, Ken, drove me home. I was relieved and glad to have the procedure done. I spent the rest of the afternoon napping on the couch in the sunshine while Ken went back to work.

Marian was not concerned. She had done what she felt she needed to do and then she rested. She had no fear or sense of danger.

🍃 Shortly after 5:00 p.m., Dr. MacColl called with the results from the biopsy. I was groggy from sleep when I answered the phone. He told me that the lump was malignant and that he wanted to see me at his office at 9:00 a.m. the next day. I agreed and then went back to sleep on the couch. When Ken came home from work, I told him what Dr. MacColl had said. Neither of us really reacted at that point. We just nodded and made a note in our calendars – Dr. MacColl, 9:00 a.m.

I look back now and wonder what I was thinking at that point. I know what "malignant" means, but somehow I just didn't associate cancer with me at that moment. I had dinner, went to bed early and had a good sleep, safe in the belief that it would be a simple matter to fix this "malignancy." When I woke the next morning, I was tense and worried but hopeful that we could easily fix this and all would be well.

It wasn't until the next day that the reality of the cancer surfaced into full consciousness – with shattering effect.

When we arrived at Dr. MacColl's office the next morning, the sun was shining and it was a beautiful prairie day. The waiting room was very crowded and I realized that Dr. Mac-Coll must have double-booked himself to fit me in on such late notice. I reminded myself to be more tolerant and patient the next time I had to wait in a doctor's office.

We were summoned to the examining room and Ken and I struggled with small talk until Dr. MacColl came into the room. He seemed unsettled and a bit disturbed. I was calm and composed. And then he told me I had "invasive lobular cancer" and would need breast surgery. I asked him if there was any chance that there could be a mistake. He was adamant. "No, there is no mistake."

My brain suddenly stopped working. As he talked, I struggled to follow the conversation. Dr. MacColl was recommending that I have a mastectomy rather than a lumpectomy. We needed to get the surgery booked right away as time was of the essence and we needed to act immediately. His nurse would prepare the consent for surgery and call for an early hospitalization date.

I was devastated. I struggled to find the questions that I knew needed to be asked and then it hit me like a bombshell that I had no idea how to proceed. All my education, all my training, all the skills that had always helped make me a good problem-solver, were puny and useless in the face of this threat. They wanted to cut off my breast and I was helpless to understand how I would ever make this decision. I was lost, frightened, disbelieving. For me the world stood still for that moment as everything in my life was swept away by a tidal wave, leaving me naked and helpless to face this unseen enemy.

Marian's dragon crept up silently and secretly while her attention was directed elsewhere. She was so involved in her day-to-day activities that she really didn't comprehend the event until it became clear that she was about to lose her breast. Like King Hrothgar, she then came face to face with the dragon's bloody footprints, and began to absorb the implications of the attack.

> We were taken to Dr. MacColl's office to sign the necessary authorizations. The nurse led me through each form, explaining the contents and pointing to the places where I needed to sign. Then she said, "This is the hardest part. This one is the consent for a mastectomy." As she said those words, I felt the enormity of what was happening to me with crushing reality and I broke down in tears. She left Ken and me alone with the promise that if I needed to change my mind later, I could do that. I don't know how long I sat at the desk with the sun streaming in the windows. I was vaguely aware of people on the other side of the glass wall going about their business – patients entering and leaving examination rooms, doctors bustling from room to room, nurses answering phones and pulling patient files. In the midst of all this normalcy, my world had been blown apart. How was I ever going to put it back together?
>
> I'm not sure what Ken's reaction was on that day. I was frozen, oblivious to what was happening around me. He held my hand and tried to comfort me as I struggled to comprehend the enormity of what was happening to me. I have never needed him more than I did at that moment and I will be forever grateful that he was there with me.

In that moment, Marian's focus shifted from outside to inside, from the bright, conscious, everyday world of business to the dark, mysterious world within. From that day on, Marian lived in a state that she called "the shadow of the dragon." For years she would be haunted by the silent, secretive raid of the "invisible enemy" within. It would become crucial for Marian to learn how to "live well in the shadow of the dragon," which meant living with mystery and the possibility of being surprised again by the invader. At the same time, Marian established a connection with her body that she did not have before. Cancer put her "on watch."

> My cancer is like an invisible enemy to me. It takes different forms depending on my mood or how I'm feeling. I never know quite how to recognize it or where it will strike. This makes it that much more frightening. Even now that I've recovered, each little ache or pain alarms me. What is that pain in my knee bone? Or the stitch in my side – has it metastasized to my bowel? Mostly, these are just the aches and pains of life, but I still analyze each sensation: is this something familiar or is this new?
>
> As time passes, I'm regaining confidence in my body and my health. With each passing day, the dragon gets a little smaller and a little farther away. It takes a long time and I feel like I must always be vigilant for the next attack. I have won a second chance at life, but it is only a reprieve. The dragon is still close by and I don't know where or when it might strike again.

Franci's cancer also crept up silently. She had paid attention to her inner sense that something wasn't right, but after the doctor told her she was too young to get a mammogram, she dismissed her concerns. It was not difficult to do. There were many things going on in her life that drew her attention outside. Her younger cousin Susie was dying of cancer. Franci had applied to transfer her airlines job from Toronto to Vancouver so that she could live closer to her family. And her brother was getting married in Calgary, so she was busy preparing to fly west.

On a hot, late summer night in 1997, Franci went to take a shower and noticed a lump on her breast. She resolved to have it checked when she returned to Toronto after the wedding. She wasn't about to mention the lump to anyone at the wedding. The family was crushed by what was happening to her cousin and the mere mention of cancer would shatter the celebratory atmosphere.

When she came back home, Franci went to the Breast Screening Centre at Mt. Sinai Hospital for an ultrasound and a needle aspiration.

It was a calm, pleasant environment. I felt dignified as I sat waiting to be called for an ultrasound/needle aspiration. The technician came, escorted me to this large room and helped me up onto the examination table. I could see two monitors. One was raised above the table [possibly for the patient's viewing] and one was behind my head, for the technician's use. As she placed the ultrasound scanner on my breast at 12 o'clock, where I felt the lump, I saw it, clear as day! The radiologist then came to do the needle aspiration. She did not have much to say, but asked me, "Why did you wait so long?"

I was rather perplexed by her question and said, "My doctor who referred me here thought it was just a cyst in need of aspirating." At that moment, sitting atop the examining table half-clothed, I sensed something was definitely not right. I didn't want to get too upset or overreact, but I didn't know really what to make of the comment. I just knew it was not very positive.

The very next day my GP phoned me and left a message on my answering machine to contact him right away.

I knew then, as soon as I heard his message. When I placed the call, his receptionist first said he was with a patient. When

I told her who was calling, she put me through to him immediately. My gut knew!

The doctor said, "Franci, the lump must come out."

I asked him, "How bad is this?"

He said it was not good news. "A tumor with abnormalities everywhere."

"Do you mean *cancer*?" I asked.

The doctor advised me that he couldn't say exactly how bad it was until they removed the tumor and did a biopsy. Still, it had to be removed, sooner rather than later. He then told me he was arranging for me to meet with a surgeon for Monday (it was Friday afternoon).

On Monday, the surgeon explained everything she possibly could and then asked me to take some time to absorb all the information she gave me. I had to phone her the next day to confirm that she told me I had breast cancer. I thought I was so strong and invincible. This news knocked the wind right out of my sails. I couldn't breathe. I had to research and learn everything I could about this disease. There I was with my mother, only two years since her diagnosis, and we were about to embark on her youngest daughter's passage through hell. A nightmare for her, her niece (my cousin) and now me. *Oh my God! What the heck was going on with our family?*

The very next day, Franci got a phone call from Vancouver saying that the airlines job was hers. She had to turn it down. In her imagery, Franci described what it felt like to come face to face at last with that green-winged fire breather that lived underground.

🌿 As one who loves the summer and the outdoors, all my leisure pursuits and activities were focused on being outside. It was a magnificent Indian summer afternoon when I came upon the dragon tracks. Immediately I froze, I could not move. All I could hear and feel was the pounding of my heart. My instant thoughts were to stay calm. I could sense the dragon slowly circling around me. Trying desperately to compose myself, the smell of the dragon's fire became more evident as the rising smoke from its nostrils was now in direct sight.

I tried to look away, but when I turned my head the dragon reached out its long neck in a straight line towards me. Now face to face, our eyes met, and in one blink of the eye the dragon released a long roar, spewing fire from deep within its belly. I fell to the ground and tried urgently to get away, but the flame captured me. I got up and ran on for what seemed like miles. I could feel myself consumed by the burning flame but did not stop moving. Eventually the fire subsided; all that surrounded me were the warm, smoldering cinders.

I looked behind to see the dragon moving on slowly and quietly in another direction, most likely in search of other prey....

RESPONSES TO THE STRIKE

When cancer appeared from out of the dark, mysterious depths of their bodies, the survivors underwent a range of responses. Some women were so engaged in outer activities and plans that they hardly acknowledged the invader. Others experienced deep shock because they saw no reason why they should have been targeted for attack. And others were so unhappy or tangled up in a web of circumstance that the cancer diagnosis seemed like a form of release.

"Not Now, I've Got Other Plans!"

For some women, cancer came at a time when they were energetically pursuing plans for the future. They portrayed their cancer as an extremely unwelcome intruder that they simply wanted out of the way. Until the dragon turned their world upside down, they were not willing to admit it was there.

Brenda Welsh and her husband, Stephen, had just purchased a new home in Toronto, and they were busy renovating it when a whole string of unexpected events occurred. Her father died rather suddenly at the age of 62 during an operation in which esophageal cancer was detected. While recovering from the shock of her father's death, she learned that her husband's company was restructuring, and Stephen had to go looking for another job.

Brenda's main dream, however, was to have a baby. For three years she and her husband had been trying to conceive a child without success. Finally, in 1996, when Brenda was in her mid-30s, the couple decided to seek professional help. Brenda went to a gynecologist who recommended that she have a laparoscopy, which established that she had endometriosis. (Endometriosis occurs when the tissue that lines the uterus grows outside the uterus and forms cysts or lesions in the pelvic cavity.) During the laparoscopy the cysts were removed and her hopes of conceiving were restored. Her fallopian tubes looked clear and everything else seemed normal.

Brenda and Stephen continued trying to conceive, but after six months without results Brenda had a sonohysterogram (an ultrasound that shows the shape of the uterine cavity). Several days prior to the test, Brenda noticed some discharge from her breast, a few drops of light brown, clear, odorless liquid. The technician who did the sonohysterogram suggested that she see her doctor. The test indicated that the uterine cavity and lining were normal, but the fallopian tubes appeared to be blocked. Brenda went back to her office in tears of frustration. She wasn't really thinking about the cancer at this point.

❧ I do remember telling a friend that I thought something was wrong; my body just did not feel right. I certainly did not think it was cancer, but something was just not right.

When she saw her GP about the breast discharge, the GP said she thought it was a breast infection and didn't think it was serious. Still, she sent Brenda for an ultrasound and Brenda complied, mainly preoccupied with the possible blockage in her fallopian tubes. After the ultrasound was done, the supervising radiologist requested that a mammogram be taken. Then, on July 2, Brenda's GP called and asked her to come in.

❧ I said that I was very busy at work and could she just tell me over the phone. When she insisted that I come to the office, I obliged. She said I appeared to have breast cancer. I was shocked. I truly thought that it must be a mistake. After that everything happened so fast. I went into autopilot.

When my GP told me that I had a pre-admission appointment for the following day with the surgeon, I started to cry. I was not crying about possibly having cancer. I was upset that this was going to interrupt my plan to have a baby. I walked back to my office feeling very drained. My feet felt heavy and I remember being extremely aware of my surroundings. I could hear the wind and sensed that it was about to rain. The walk took about three minutes, but it felt like an eternity. I closed my office door and called my husband. As soon as I heard his voice, I started to cry. I could barely say the words. He kept asking me to speak slowly as he could not understand me. He asked me to meet him at home. After I hung up the phone, I composed myself and spoke to my supervisor. I gathered up my things and took lots of paperwork home. I knew that I would be away from the office for a while and I did not want to leave things unfinished.

Brenda and Stephen went together for her appointment with the surgeon. Brenda was still focused on the possible blockage in her fallopian tubes, and she asked the surgeon if he could check her tubes during the surgery.

🍃 When he said it was not possible, I started to feel that I was losing control. I was in the hospital much longer than I expected as they were making arrangements to have the surgery the following week. I felt impatient, as I was late for an appointment with my fertility specialist. I kept watching the time and asked Stephen to go to my fertility doctor's office to tell him that I would be late. Stephen obliged, but he did not want to leave. He must have thought that I was losing my mind. He was very concerned about the upcoming surgery and there I was, preoccupied with the news of the blockage in my fallopian tubes.

Later, while running to the office of her fertility doctor, which was down the street from the hospital, Brenda told herself that the breast cancer could still be a mistake. She would proceed with her plan to have a baby – she had come too far to let go of her dream.

🍃 I recall calmly telling the fertility doctor about my upcoming surgery. I felt emotionless. I asked if he could come to the hospital while I was having the mastectomy to check the fallopian tubes.

He said, "You need to focus all your energy on beating the cancer." That was the first time that I thought that maybe it was true, I really did have breast cancer. I felt rather panicky. I asked him if he could freeze some of my eggs. No, not a good idea. I would need to take hormones to get the eggs to multiply and that was too dangerous with my current diagnosis of breast cancer. I remember fighting back the tears and feeling a sense of sadness. He suggested that I read the books *The Art of Chi Kung* and *Mastering Miracles*.

When we got home, Stephen was visibly shaken. It was one of the few times I have ever seen my husband in this state. He was sitting on the sofa and I could not understand why he was so upset. He could not understand why I was calmly doing my paperwork.

I worked that night until around 8:00 p.m. It was strange, but I felt extremely focused on my work. I just had a need to get my paperwork done. It was like I was putting my affairs in order. Dying was certainly not on my mind, but maybe subconsciously I was thinking about it.

Later, I got a second opinion about harvesting the eggs. This fertility specialist asked me to think about what would happen if we harvested the eggs and then I died. "What would you want done with the eggs?" she asked. I thought that was a strange question. I was frustrated that she was questioning my mortality.

Just prior to surgery, the surgeon came to speak to me. I was sitting in the waiting room, clutching a pillow, wearing my blue hospital gown, cap and paper slippers. I asked him, "Could it possibly be a mistake?"

He said, "I would not put you through all this if I thought it was a mistake." He was 99 percent sure that he would have to remove my entire breast. I felt so sad. I sat there shivering; it was extremely cold in the waiting area. A few tears dropped down my cheeks. When I lay on the operating table, I was still crying softly. A nurse asked me, "Is this the first time you have had surgery?" I shook my head no. I could not speak for fear of really starting to cry. That was the first time I realized I was about to lose my breast.

"Why Me?"

Those survivors who were most shocked could not fathom how the cancer could have happened to them. The attack was irrational, mysterious, inexplicable. They had been taking care of themselves. They were too young. Or, like Anita Ewart, they should have known better. As a diagnostic and screening mammographer, it was Anita's *job* to detect cancer.

Prior to her diagnosis, Anita was living in Prince George, B.C., and working as a mammographer. At the age of 49, she had just resigned from the Canadian Cancer Society as an educator and facilitator of a "Living with Cancer" support group. Anita was tired and stressed and she was rapidly reaching burnout. She was definitely not prepared for a cancer diagnosis. It left her completely mystified.

It all started when she went to her surgeon to drain a tiny axillary lump and he couldn't get any fluid.

> I knew in my gut that this boded *bad* and felt instantly nauseous. I could smell fear. My ears buzzed and I don't recall any of his words other than "biopsy for the suspicious calcifications from your screening exam" and "will have a look at *this* too." The cancer was diagnosed through open biopsy – the lump was an "infiltrating ductile carcinoma."
>
> When my GP told me, I swore like some deranged subhuman and cried: "Why *me*? I work as a mammographer, for heaven's sake. I do regular breast self-examinations. I *had* the lump checked out five months ago! There's no family history – none. What have I done to deserve this? *Why? What?*" I cried, over and over. Somehow I got back to the x-ray department and collapsed in tears in the darkroom with all my staff around, stunned.

Here's how Anita portrayed her dragon:

The dragon was black in color, dangerous, very threatening and huge. It lived secretly, hidden away, but was perhaps lurking in my subconscious. Had I perhaps imagined its presence before? It struck with little warning, although I may have been slightly prewarned by the biopsy I had the year before in '94. It surprised me, shocked me out of my boots. I spent agonizing hours trying to figure out *why*.

Anita continued to be plagued by the question "Why me?" for which she had no answers, until one day, when another question occurred to her: "Why *not* me?"

"I'm Almost Relieved"

At other times, the women's worlds were so chaotic that the dragon's strike was almost, in a strange way, welcome. When she found out she had cancer, Barb Chomski of Toronto was a 44-year-old working mom, single, and single-handedly trying to support twin teenage girls and an 11-year-old son.

Before I got diagnosed, my life was a whirlwind. I was in constant motion. I had a lot of stress in my life as single mom to three kids, working at a dead-end job as a waitress and feeling that my life was hanging by a thread. I ran constantly throughout my waking days, I couldn't take time off and I couldn't let anyone down. Life as a single mom with three kids was a juggling act.

Several years before her diagnosis, Barb had wrestled her way free from a violently abusive relationship with her husband of 18 years.

It wasn't all that bad at the beginning, but progressively he got worse. We all believed that there was something wrong with him mentally, but he wouldn't go and get help. So his mental condition deteriorated. He took it out on me, physically and mentally. Near the end it was really bad. I tried to get a restraining order against him. I couldn't get him to leave the house. So I kept leaving with the kids and going to my mom's or my sister's, and meanwhile I tried to live, to work, take the kids to school... I tried to function like a normal person.

Finally I realized that he was going to kill me if something didn't happen. After different types of arrests (he would stalk me and break into the house) we went to court, and I got him out of the house.

Over the next two years, Barb restored a sense of order in her home. She took on two jobs and worked furiously to create a normal environment for her children. Meanwhile, rest – which she sorely needed – seemed inconceivable. During that time Barb met another man and when the relationship began to get serious, he wanted to move in. Barb's kids didn't like him and so Barb resisted. Then one night while she was working in the restaurant, Barb saw him with another woman. She was heartbroken. The very next day, on Halloween of 1996, Barb discovered the lump on her breast. She had already booked a routine physical, and when the lump was checked out the doctor told her, "I'm afraid the news isn't good." Barb's worst suspicions were confirmed – but her reaction surprised her.

🌿 I don't remember thinking that I was going to die. The strongest thought in the back of my mind was that I would have to take time off work. I felt elated that now I had a legitimate reason for resting, that I would be taken care of by other people. It took something as drastic as the diagnosis of cancer for me to cut myself some slack, to put my needs ahead of others, I think that I had some emotional issues to deal with!

Among those survivors who experienced their cancer as a deadly dragon, there were a variety of initial responses to the primary "attack." Some, like Marian and Brenda Welsh, viewed the dragon as an incomprehensible, deadly enemy that shattered their lives; while others, in spite of their shock and horror, were almost relieved to have their worlds destroyed.

In *How We Die*, Dr. Sherwin B. Nuland gives a chilling description of how cancer operates – one which could be easily mistaken for a description of Grendel himself. Cancer, he writes, is "in fact berserk with the malicious exuberance of killing. The disease pursues a continual, uninhibited, circumferential, barn-burning expedition of destructiveness, in which it heeds no rules, follows no commands, and explodes all resistance in a homicidal riot of devastation." Even its origins resemble those of Grendel, who was banished by the Creator to the underworld along with all the other monsters, giants and misshapen children of Cain. The first cells of cancer are the bastard offspring of unsuspecting parent cells "who ultimately reject them because they are ugly, deformed, and unruly," writes Dr. Nuland. "In the community of living tissues, the uncontrolled mob of misfits that is cancer behaves like a gang of perpetually wilding adolescents. They are the juvenile delinquents of cellular society."

When they discovered the dragon that was loose inside their own bodies, the women were thrown into a state of numb disbelief. Like the King, they sat "stricken and helpless, bewildered and stunned, staring aghast at the demon's trail." It would take time to absorb the extent of the damage, for the dragon had, in one moment, permanently changed their lives.

II

Wounds of the Dragon

Grendel's first raid is only the beginning of a dark chapter in the reign of King Hrothgar. With his appetite for human blood whetted, the dragon keeps coming back to terrorize the neighborhood. Over and over, he attacks indiscriminately, killing the young and the old. No one can predict where he will strike next, nor can anyone stop the rampage. The once lively Hall is soon deserted, and the kingdom falls into darkness, silenced by the grim invader who prowls the moors.

The people can find no refuge, neither in the King's Hall nor in their homes, and while they brood and lie awake in their beds, the King agonizes over his powerlessness to protect his country from the malignant beast.

RUNNING AWAY

Many of the survivors described the first few days after diagnosis as a twilight zone, a nightmare, a time when they fled the presence of the dragon. Terror was fierce and denial was strong. In 1997, when Fran Weiss discovered that she had cancer, it was easy for her to ignore because it was only one of many crises. The waters of the Red River near her home in Winnipeg were rising. Her neighbors were losing their homes. Her brother announced he had AIDS. As a registered nurse and mother of six, Fran had a lot of other people to be concerned about.

For a while she ran around attending to other calamities, hoping that after her lumpectomy the cancer would be shown to be intra-ductal (i.e., there were too many cells in the ducts of the tissue, which is not a serious problem). Unfortunately, the cancer was invasive – small (only six millimeters in size) but aggressive. As Fran said of the wound her dragon inflicted: "It was not a little white poodle of a family pet, but a brute of a Rottweiler attack."

> My beloved little brother was fatally ill. The Red River was rising, threatening Winnipeg with the flood of the century. Our home is within a block of the river. Sandbagging was in progress. The whole world was falling apart simultaneously – the flood, my brother and myself. The river was an omi-nous presence at all times, because it was around us in terms of sandbags, army camps down the street, headlines in the newspapers. There was no calm, no peace anywhere, no refuge.

Gone were the days of taking nice, quiet walks along the river-bank. Now when she went outside, Fran saw sandbags piled up everywhere, and her head teemed with worries over the safety of neighbors and what her family would do if the sewers backed up. Fran also felt guilty because she couldn't take anyone into her home. It was no longer a safe place – it too could be flooded. Nor was she in a state to be hospitable. With all these events occupying her concerns, Fran didn't focus on her cancer until she went to the oncology clinic at St. Boniface Hospital.

> It was on registering there that I really came to the deep, depressing appreciation that I had cancer, and would be deeply embroiled with the medical system for a long, *long* time. On arrival, one is welcomed warmly and compassion-

ately, and *registered*. They took my photograph. This was the final straw. I was cornered!

My workplace at that time was a long-term care facility. The first thing we did when we received a new resident was welcome them and take their photograph. To me, there always seemed something sad and permanent about that snapshot. One is *in* the system. There is no escaping. One's options and freedoms have greatly diminished. One is captured. One is almost not an individual any more. Those in charge have seen so many of you, they probably won't remember your face without a photographic reference.

Fran was cornered. There was no other way to go but *through*.

Loss of Innocence and Security

After Grendel attacked, the world of the people in Hrothgar's kingdom changed forever. They could no longer go outside without fear; they could no longer celebrate with the carefree abandon of those who are assured of the King's protection. Many survivors of breast cancer experienced that painful loss of security. When she was asked what the dragon took from her, Julie Dubuc of Winnipeg said:

> The dragon I met was very cunning and had the ability to make himself invisible when it suited him. The dragon stole the "philosopher's stone" from me. The stone is a magical substance that only the young, healthy and innocent can own. It offers a cloak that the user can wear to guard against death and promises immortality to those who believe in it.

In medieval alchemy, the philosopher's stone was believed to have had the magical power to transform corruptible metals into gold. Until she was diagnosed with cancer, Julie enjoyed the youthful illusion that she was immortal and invincible. She didn't know she possessed the philosopher's stone until the dragon came along, stole it and stripped her of the insulating illusion. Like the people in *Beowulf*, she was suddenly exposed to the reality of disease and death. The dragon could spring out from the shadows at any time, in any place.

Chantal Brunet, who lives in Montreal, was only 30 when she was diagnosed. She described her dragon as a creature who slept peacefully in its cave until, in her 20s, Chantal began to feel unhappy in her marriage. Sensing her distress, the dragon grew restless and disturbed. When she was diagnosed with cancer, her dragon came out of the cave and "struck like lightning," destroying the cheerful green fields of her childhood. Her world fell into darkness – beauty fled, youth fled, love fled.

> My mind cannot see the beauty any more. Where did the beauty go? My mind is in complete darkness. I look at myself in the pond and I cannot even recognize myself. This *isn't* me! I used to be so beautiful! Is it my mind, or my imagination? Maybe it is reality. Maybe... Oh! The sky! It's suddenly overcast. The sky is closing up on me. Hey! Blue sky! Where are you going? Wait for me! Wait! Come back! I am *begging* you, please don't go, don't go, don't leave me all alone, by myself, with no umbrella to protect me.... I need you. I need someone to hold my hand. I need your warmth, please, I am *begging* you!
>
> I am crying in my soul. There, in the middle of the field, I see no more flowers. No more children are laughing – they don't come around any more. It is not fun to play here any longer. It is so depressing. The air is gray, the grass is yellowish,

like after winter, as if it is dying out. The birds have died and
they lie here, next to the big tree, next to me. So many birds,
so much pain, so many deaths. Why? I don't know. And I can't
help it. Well, I can. But I have no strength.

I am lying on my side, my body completely on the ground.
I can't get up – the weight of my pain is keeping me down.
I have tears rolling silently down on my cheeks, the roll of
desperation. I am shaking… I'm cold and I'm scared. Feeling
lonely. Feeling so lonely. I finally fall asleep with the rain
falling on my body and the lightning and thunder breaking up
the sky. I cannot even see the moon any more. The sky has
closed up on me.

The cancer diagnosis cast a long shadow over the survivors'
worlds. It robbed them of their innocence, threw their immediate
world into turmoil, and darkened their hopes for the future. As
Anita said:

🌿 The hardest loss was losing my long-time dream of living to
a ripe old age. Women on both sides of my family lived *long*
lives, like 88, 92, 94, 90 and almost (two weeks short of) 101!
What the *hell* was I doing facing possible death at the age of
49? I had to leave behind the youthful vision of immortality.
Suddenly my inevitable mortality was slammed in my face,
and I hated that. I wasn't ready to even think about it, let
alone *deal* with it.

Loss of Power and Control

On first impact, most women received the diagnosis as a "death sentence." Like the King in *Beowulf*, they were stunned by the unexpected attack and bewildered by their powerlessness to do anything about it. Those who had been strong managers and rulers of their own domain were often the ones most thrown off guard when their sense of control was suddenly undermined.

For Evelyn Crofts, one slip on the carpet and she slid off the edge of the world. Evelyn worked as an administrative assistant for the city council of Newmarket, Ontario, and she had a nine-year-old daughter and a new husband. Prior to her cancer diagnosis in 1994 she had endured 10 years of "unbearable stress" during which time she had separated and divorced; her brother, her father and her ex-husband had all passed away; and, throughout, she had held on to a very demanding job. At last she remarried and had a baby.

🌿 At 40 my life had started to settle down, but not before it was to come crashing down.

I was cleaning and slipped backwards on an area rug. I went to the floor straight on my back. I don't remember a lot about that fateful day, but I do remember that I fell hard. It was a moment in time that changed everything, but was it a curse or was it a blessing? Only time would tell.

My back was so sore that I wanted to lie down, so I did, but when I tried to get up, I couldn't. It took a lot of fancy maneuvering before I was able to sit on the side of the bed. My doctor's office was a few miles away, so I decided to go to my husband's doctor, whose office was nearby. An x-ray was taken and it was felt that I had pneumonia. I was sent home to bed with the appropriate medicine. I had never had pneumonia so I wasn't sure just how I was supposed to feel, but after a couple of days, when I still couldn't pull myself up out of the bed, I began to think that perhaps that diagnosis wasn't right. So this time I made an appointment with my own doctor.

He decided to send me for a bone scan. A few days later I'm called to go to his office at about 7:00 p.m. I walk into my doctor's office, and I notice that there are no other patients there except me. I immediately get this sinking feeling. This is an office that is usually triple-booked. At any given time you wait at least an hour before you can see the doctor. I'm called in and my doctor proceeds to tell me about these hot spots on the bone scan, but he doesn't say the "c" word. It doesn't matter because I know what it means – I know – I know – I know. Finally, as the doctor is examining me, he mentions the "c" word. He says that the hot spots are the secondary cancer in my bones, and that they need to find the primary. I tell him that I think the primary cancer is in the breasts. After all, my mother's two sisters had breast cancer: one lived – one died.

I reacted to the diagnosis with stunned wonder. This year was to be the turning point in my life. This was the year I turned 40. This was the year that I had my first mammogram and everything was supposed to be okay. How can this be? It was all so surreal.

I got in my van to drive home. I was almost home before I realized that the interior light was on in the van. I couldn't get myself to go home. How could I tell my husband? How were we going to tell my nine-year-old daughter? How was I, the youngest child of four, going to tell my aging mother who had already lost one child? *I couldn't go home with the diagnosis, I just couldn't.* I stopped at a telephone booth and gave my husband the dreadful news. He came to the booth, and he was able to get me to come home.

Evelyn was given 18 months to live. All of a sudden she faced a whirlwind of choices about what treatment to seek, where and how. The new life she had won through so much hardship had been senselessly overthrown in an instant.

〰 Without a doubt, the hardest loss of all, both physically and psychologically, at least to me, was the loss of control. They could cut my hair, they could cut my body parts, but to take away my ability to be in control of my life was unbearably painful. I felt that everything was slipping away, little by little.

Early in my diagnosis, I remember sitting in one of the many hospitals that was soon to become like a second home to me, and I saw an elderly person with one of his limbs missing. I remember thinking, *If only I were here for the same reason that person is here, I could at least live with one leg.* You think very different thoughts. Some thoughts are very selfish, and some thoughts are just the opposite. I remember picking out special songs for the people in my life that meant the most to me.

Cancer treatment changes one's physical appearance, and in most cases not for the better. However, I have found that the physical loss is pale in comparison to the psychological loss. I know many women with plenty of battle scars, and it is truly amazing what these women endure, but their emotional scars are much less visible. The anxiety is, at times, overwhelming.

For Evelyn, the deepest wound of breast cancer was the anxiety of being exposed to death without the power to do anything about it. Many women shared this emotional wound. Cancer weakened and bewildered them, causing them to walk around in a state of constant unease and vigilance, terrified of shadows.

At times the people who suffered the greatest loss of control were not the women but their husbands or partners. When Bernice Kwasnicki of Winnipeg was diagnosed at the age of 53, her husband would not speak to her about the disease. Cancer forced Bernice to make decisions on her own behalf, for her own survival, and it put her out of reach of her husband.

〰 My husband felt that this disease had taken control over me. Still, he was the one who helped me the most with everyday care – with my bandages, bathing, dressing, preparing meals, keeping the house tidy, and driving me back and forth to medical appointments. He would even lie in the same position all night just so I could prop my arm on him and get some sleep.

All this, but he would not talk about cancer. He tuned me out if I tried to express my feelings on the subject. I found this to be a very lonesome situation. I had our daughters, my sisters, my mother and my friends to talk to, but it was his conversation that I wanted and needed to hear so badly. I felt hurt by his behavior.

Three years later, I've developed a mild case of lymphedema in my left arm/back areas. It's not so great, but I've learned to keep it under control with the help of a physiotherapist.

My husband's hands help me alleviate some of the pressure due to fluid retention. He rubs my arm and back ever so softly, coaxing the lymphatic system to do its work. Still, he holds out – no conversation about cancer. I think he feels this is at least a small bit of control he still has. He knows I would love to hear some positive views about what has happened these past three years.

When Bernice reflected on why her husband suffered such a deep loss of control, she remembered the painful experience he had undergone when, at the age of 15, his mother died and he witnessed his father's grief.

🌿 He saw his father walk around the perimeter of the farm, howling at the top of his head, mourning his wife. It stayed with him. So when I got cancer I felt for him because I knew he was thinking, *Oh, I'm going to relive my past.* But I couldn't help him, I had to help me. I had to get better, I had to get strong.

Cancer exposed the women to the possibility of death, and it exposed their families too. Like the King in *Beowulf*, some survivors worried over the fate of the women in their families. Bernice, who had no previous family history of breast cancer, felt guilty about bringing the disease into the household.

The diagnosis meant that I had caused all the females in my family to be more concerned about their mortality, now that cancer was a factor in mine. Being the eldest of nine children, seven of us being women – each with families where women predominate – made me feel so much more regretful. I felt so guilty for bringing this demon into the lives of our daughters and grandchildren. I knew that I must fight all that much harder to show them there is life after diagnosis.

LOSS OF TRUST

Some women said that the hardest loss to deal with was the loss of trust. Cancer set them at odds with the bodies they had once relied upon to carry them through life. They were alarmed to discover that their bodies were no longer a safe haven, and to some this seemed like a deep and confounding betrayal. Cathy Prusak, a good-natured Winnipeg pharmacist who had always been self-confident and, in her husband's words, "smart as a whip," was completely unprepared for the news of her cancer. Until she reached her early 30s, she had taken her health for granted.

🌿 I was generally caught up in the rat race. I would come home from long days at work and flake out on the couch. Self-care was definitely not a word in my vocabulary. I had good relationships with my family and friends, but perhaps took a lot of that for granted. Looking back now, I don't see that I took the time out to nurture the relationships that were important in my life, nor did I really think about what was essential to my survival. My life was picture perfect looking in, but looking back I would say it was less than complete.

Cathy's life changed the moment her surgeon read her the pathology report from her biopsy.

🌿 As she read the report, I felt as though I was being kicked in the head. Since the first mammogram I had been reassured that the lump was likely nothing. What she read was definitely not nothing. It was a collection of scary words including "invasive," which stood out particularly in my mind. I was being invaded!

I accepted the news quite calmly and said thank you as I left her office with requisitions in my hand. I went to the lab for some blood work. Standing at the lab was the most surreal moment in the whole diagnostic journey. I couldn't reconcile the fact that my name was on a requisition with the words "Breast CA" in the diagnosis box. I wanted to erase it.

I had gone to the ill-fated appointment by myself, so I proceeded to drive myself home. I'm not really sure how I got home, or if I killed anyone along the way. It was a bit of a blur. After getting home I proceeded to call my husband at work. What happened to me at that point was again completely surreal and out of character for me. I couldn't speak, literally. Marc answered the phone at work, and all I could do was sort of whine and snort. He recognized my voice, although I don't know how because I didn't come close to forming any intelligible words. He knew what I was trying to tell him and came straight home. That moment was very disturbing to me. I couldn't believe that I was so weak, that this had jolted me so badly.

Cathy's description of her dragon expressed her feeling of being suddenly and unexpectedly betrayed.

 My dragon was very sinister and sneaky. I don't have a clue what it looked like, because I didn't see it coming. It struck so fast and unexpectedly and I didn't get a good look at it even then.

Brenda Tierney from Burnaby, B.C., also felt that her body had betrayed her. Brenda had lived a healthy life; there was no cause for the disease. She had just completed her accounting designation and she was slowly building up her practice. She and her 16-year-old son had started to travel. She didn't fit the breast cancer profile. She had taken good care of herself, she had tried to lead a balanced life, and it hadn't worked.

Even her diagnosis had an air of unreality about it. She found the cancer herself – and persisted in getting a clear diagnosis even though the doctor didn't think she needed to be concerned.

 For some reason I chose to pursue the small thickening in my breast. No one took me too seriously because I didn't fit into the statistical profile of a person who was supposed to get cancer. Although "something" was detected on an ultrasound, I was told to come back in three months. When I finally saw a doctor who could do a biopsy, he wasn't sure whether I should have one or not. I finally said to him, "If I were your wife, what would you do?"

This statement seemed to make him pause, and he said, "Well, I'd recommend she have a biopsy."

So I said, "I want one."

After the biopsy had been done, Brenda's GP received a letter from the specialist saying that Brenda was probably okay, but he didn't have the actual results because of a strike at the University of British Columbia. Brenda asked her GP to phone the university and get the results.

🍂 He seemed quite annoyed at my persistence. I went home. While I was trying to unlock the door, I could hear the telephone ringing. The results were not what had been expected; the growth was malignant and invasive.

I just couldn't believe that there was a possibility that this was going to be the end of my life. I didn't have the energy to talk. At times I was hysterical. At one point I remember screaming, "I don't want to die!" Life seemed so black.

Brenda was boggled by the mystery of why cancer had invaded her, and was deeply offended by the suggestion that she had done something to cause her illness.

🍂 The hardest loss of all was my loss of confidence in my body. I hated the thought that I was sick. I didn't know what else I could do and I was afraid of reoccurrence. In 1989, some of the professionals such as doctors, nutritionists and psychologists indicated that getting cancer was your own fault, and this made me feel guilty as well as angry.

Loss of Femininity

When the dragon entered the women's lives, it not only robbed them of innocence, security, power and trust, it also hurt them deeply and personally. It forced them to relinquish parts of themselves that were crucial to their identity as women and mothers – and nowhere was that loss more excruciating than in the loss of their breasts.

The loss of breasts, and the scars that lingered from the surgery, dealt a major blow to the survivors' self-image, not to mention their relationships, their sex lives and their fertility. The wound cut to the core of their identity and stripped them of the pride and joy they had taken in their bodies. For young, single women, the loss of breasts sometimes had a shattering impact on their sense of femininity and on their relationships.

Chantal, an attractive woman with dark hair and eyes, was only 30 when she was diagnosed. After struggling with an unhappy marriage, she had separated from her husband and divorced in 1994. Right after the divorce she began to date another man. After two months of dating, Chantal and her four-year-old son moved in with the new boyfriend. From the beginning, she knew it was a mistake.

🖋 Typical cliché, divorce and rematch! It was wrong to move in, and I knew it. I was unhappy in my love life and I was unhappy with myself, but I was petrified to be alone.

In August of 1995, Chantal found a lump on her breast while in the shower. She had no family history of breast cancer, so the oncologist told her just to watch it for a little while. It was still there after three months and so Chantal had a biopsy, which showed a malignant tumor on her right breast.

〰 The doctor called me at home asking me to come the next day because I had "abnormal" cells. I hung up the phone and I panicked. I realized that the worst thing that can happen to a woman is breast cancer. Although I was not certain that it was cancer, I surely did not like the idea of having "abnormal" cells. I imagined the worst. And it happened.

Overwhelmed by fear and panic, Chantal went down to the hospital the next day, and before she knew it, she had signed the forms authorizing her surgeon to remove her breast.

〰 One week later, on Valentine's Day, February 14, 1996, bang! I was operated on and my breast was removed. Happy Valentine's!

Chantal said her boyfriend did not lay a hand on her after the operation. "He was turned off." Nor did he become any more supportive when she went through chemo.

〰 He would come with me to the hospital and there he would flirt with a gorgeous redhead while I was hooked up on intravenous for my treatment. Or he would fall asleep. What a jerk! At home, he would leave me and go downstairs to do whatever. It was too much for him to handle.

I made a choice to confront him with the situation. On May 1, shortly before my last chemo treatment, I moved out and went to live with my brother. That was the best decision I ever made. I was losing my soul, my heart, my values. And my poor son! He was so young, only four years old, and there I was with a bald Kojak head.

While Chantal suffered the losses of her breast, her hair and her feelings of femininity, nothing was as painful as the wound of rejection. She became hostile towards men.

🖋 I thought that men were all a bunch of selfish, body-oriented, inconsiderate and weak human beings. I turned away even the men who were interested and didn't care about me having one breast. I went from relationship to relationship just to make sure I could keep my emotional wound wide open. I did not believe my friends (or my brother) when they told me that the "right" man would accept me the way I am.

Chantal couldn't accept herself as she was; she could not meet her own image in the mirror.

🖋 For at least two years after, when I looked in the mirror, I focused on each little inch of my unperfect body. It is funny in a way. I was "accepting" (so I thought) my flat chest, but I was constantly complaining about my stomach, my legs, arms or anything that bothered me. And of course, once in a while I would all of a sudden "wake up" and burst into tears, crying over my ugly, deteriorating, aging body.

With the loss of her breast, Chantal felt that she had lost the power of her femininity – the one thing she had relied upon for her happiness and self-esteem.

🖋 Breasts! Beautiful woman's breasts! Isn't this part of any woman's aura of femininity? Kind of a power we possess. A power of seduction. The power of a mother. You don't have to show them off to feel that power. And you don't need to wear sexy blouses to feel it either.

No. Breasts will feed a child, breasts will be part of sexual desire, breasts will make a simple dress look so sexy, and breasts in a beautiful bra make a true piece of art.

So, if you don't like your legs, and you don't like your tummy, you can say to yourself while looking in the mirror, *Thank God I'm beautiful from the waist up!* That's how I felt before the cancer. I felt like a woman, with beautiful breasts and a pretty face (but I hated the rest of my body).

For some time Chantal lived in a state of complete dejection. Her femininity had been ruined and would never come back; she felt she had lost all chance for a happy life. "I was finished," she said.

Sadly, Chantal was not alone in being rejected by her partner. It was a story several women told. Their abandonment left them wondering if anyone would love them. And yet, through the loss, they began to discover what true femininity, identity and friendship meant. Pamela Robbins, who lives by the water at Halfmoon Bay in British Columbia, was also abandoned by her partner. Today, she boisterously describes herself as an "ex-teacher, age 52, and flat-chested!"

Pamela's journey with breast cancer began back in 1975, when doctors found a pre-cancerous condition in her breasts. It led to a series of lumpectomies, a slow cutting away at her breasts. Then, while she was in Australia in 1998, Pamela and a friend witnessed a breast cancer event that had ominous overtones for both women.

〰 While in Canberra visiting a long-time girlfriend, I was struck by a powerful display on the lawn in front of Parliament House. Hundreds of hot pink paper dolls stood in the shape of a woman, representing women diagnosed each year with breast cancer in Australia. They were surrounded by white dolls representing the women who die. Not only was I deeply moved but, ironically, both myself and my friend unknowingly had breast cancer at that moment, only to be diagnosed soon afterwards.

After she returned to Canada in April 1999, Pamela had a partial mastectomy and cancer was found. The partial was followed by a double mastectomy in November 1999. Then came the final blow.

My life partner was a forensic pathologist who, in order to cope with his work, could be very disconnected emotionally. After my partial mastectomy, he simply left. Three months later he returned with many apologies and promises, only to detach again after another lumpectomy and my double mastectomy. I was devastated, as I had decided to trust again.

When I found myself on my own, I got panicky thoughts. *How do I find strength to carry on alone without my partner? Who will be with me when I am feeling vulnerable and fragile after the surgery? What if I had breasts, would he have stayed? Will anyone else want me now that I don't have breasts? Will I find someone to love* me *as I am?*

These were huge losses for me, both physically and psychologically. I felt a big empty space on my chest right over the big hole I felt in my heart.

Nor did Pamela get much support from her family. Like her partner, she says, her family was also "emotionally disconnected," unable to deal with feelings or issues.

During my breast cancer ordeal, I was told I was "making a mountain out of a molehill" and "whining." I became very enlightened about what it means to be supportive. Some friends were very supportive and helpful; others were disinterested or trivialized my surgeries with statements like, "Oh well, who needs breasts anyway." (Well, I don't need them, but they are body parts.) Or, "Be thankful it's not an arm." (of course I am, thank you.) Or, "Be positive." (More a plea to be so for them, not for me.)

These collective losses were too much to grieve, so I just went into shock until I was ready to deal with them, bit by bit.

The single young women who told their stories to us were

particularly sensitive about new relationships, and many had not pursued them. They weren't ready – cancer took them into a kind of cocoon. Barb Chomski didn't know how she would broach the subject of breast cancer with an intimate new friend.

⚘ I haven't had intimate relationships since the cancer. I feel … I don't know, something's changed. Weight gain came with the chemo – that altered me physically – and I lost a lot of hair. But I seemed to cocoon myself. I surrounded myself with my friends and family. I really didn't feel attractive, so I wasn't looking. I thought, *Who would look at me anyway?*

Again, I'm thinking if I start a new relationship, someone brand new, do I tell them? How do I tell them? It's very different. I don't know what I'm going to do about that. If it happens, it happens, I guess. If it's meant to be. I'm not lonely or anything. I've had so much trouble with men, maybe I'm better off without them. I call myself a recycled virgin!

Franci felt the same way:

⚘ I have gone on dates, but I haven't met anyone special enough to share myself with, never mind my story. It would have to be someone very genuine. Cancer does take away your femininity. Not that I'm totally disfigured or deformed – I'm lucky. But I have a big scar – it's noticeable. A part of me is gone. I don't know if I've reconciled that yet.

One day, while she was at work, Franci was surprised to hear what a man might think about the loss of a woman's breasts.

⚘ One of the men at work made a funny statement that took me aback at first. We were having coffee, we weren't close or anything. He had been talking about somebody in his family who had gone through cancer and surgery. Then suddenly he said, "Franci, don't worry about it. *Tits are for kids.*"

I was shocked! I had never discussed my situation with him and I guess he was thinking I had a mastectomy. But I thought about it. Until you're affected by something like this you feel whole and beautiful, you have a youthful outlook on life. I still have a positive outlook, but cancer took away my innocence, a part of my childhood. Any guy who focuses on breasts and not the person isn't the guy for me.

So I said to him, "You know, you're right. Tits *are* for kids."

The loss or scarring of their breasts affected the women's husbands and partners too. The most loving and sensitive husband could still be floored by the news that his spouse was going to lose her breasts. Akky Mansikka, a special education teacher in Toronto, had large breasts, and when she and her husband came to the doctor's office to hear the report following her needle biopsy, neither of them were prepared for the news. The doctor said he had definitely found cancer and there were signs that the cancer was present in both breasts. He recommended a double mastectomy.

Reality hit like a punch in the stomach. Life seemed to stop right there. Henry was so shocked, he *passed out.* He slid out of his chair and onto the floor. A few minutes later he came to, thinking it was a bad nightmare, and said, "I thought he said a double mastectomy!" I said, "Yes, he did," and he *passed out again!* For an hour he lay there being treated and looked after in the examining room. The nurse brought him water and the doctor came in to check on him occasionally. The doctor was in a rush and didn't have time to deal with me. I kept thinking, *What about me?*

Some partners were very sensitive and there were moments of great intimacy in the loss. Anita felt that her husband was her most important helper in many ways.

He would say things like, "I'd rather love you alive with one breast than dead with both of them." And, "Let's not worry until we *have* to."

On an intimate note, he was respectful of my undressing in the dark. He was protective and understanding. He listened. And listened. And listened. God, but he's a patient man. He never really looked at the scar until I made him. I had to see if it repulsed him, but he didn't let me down, even then. His face never changed, except that he smiled and told me I had to put on some weight because now my ribs were showing. I thank God every day for having such a supportive partner. I know too many women who have been abandoned physically, emotionally and sexually after a mastectomy, and that fact sickens me. It disgusts my husband as well.

For the women who were finished child-rearing, the loss of breasts was often associated with the loss of motherhood. When Akky lost her breasts at the age of 50, she felt as though she had come to the end of her life. The mastectomy precipitated a farewell to her fertile years, her nurturing identity. Her children had grown up and were leaving home. She felt invisible and unrecognized at home and at work, and yet powerless to make changes in her life. On some level the cancer diagnosis didn't come as a surprise. As Akky said, "It almost seemed like a way out." With the loss of her breasts, Akky lost her identity as a mother, and with it, her bearings and direction in life.

In the week after I got home from the hospital, I kept having nightmares about losing things, especially pairs of things. It started in my nightmares with a life-and-death search for a pair of missing candelabras. I had to find them. I was obsessed by finding them. They were so important to me. I had never realized how important they were because I never put great value on such things; after all, they were just ornaments to decorate a table. I never appreciated how beautiful they were, so shiny and silver. They had such beautiful gentle curves and added so much grace and elegance to the dining-room table and to the home in general. They were a family heirloom and so valuable. They were irreplaceable. The nightmares continued with other missing things, and in one nightmare I went searching in a nearby shopping mall for my twin toddlers that had gone missing. It occurred to me the nightmares were about losses – pairs of losses – breasts. Henry, my husband, finally commented, "I think the missing things are your boobs."

The nightmares cleared up after that. It was very sad for me, even though I had two lovely new man-made ones. I would no longer be able to nurse my children. I could no longer be a nurturer, a mother. Although we had not planned to have any more children, the choices were gone. When I lost my breasts, I realized that my youth was gone as well as beauty. It seemed the essence of being female was gone. Everything society values in females – youth, beauty, motherhood – all gone. Everything I thought I valued was gone, but then, I had never given such things much thought until I was diagnosed and had a double mastectomy.

Brenda Welsh's most cherished dream was to have her own baby, and she lost her fertility to cancer. After her mastectomy, the oncologist informed her that she had stage III breast cancer. An aggressive treatment plan of chemotherapy and radiation was recommended. Doctors explained to her that they hoped to kill any trace of cancer left in her body, but to Brenda that also meant killing the chance of ever conceiving her own child.

🌿 I recall starting to feel rather dizzy. I asked, in a state of tears, if I could possibly focus on conceiving first, and after I had my baby I would start the therapy. The doctor explained that a pregnancy for me could cause the cancer to spread. My husband, Stephen, was with me at the appointment. He fully supported Dr. Blondell's recommendation to proceed with the aggressive chemotherapy.

I remember feeling frustrated and angry. I wanted this to be my decision. I remember leaving the office and saying that I had to think about it. I recall being on the highway going up to the cottage. I started to sob uncontrollably. I could sense Stephen's feeling of helplessness. This was the first time I cried to such depth. I felt trapped. I remember Stephen saying he wanted me around more than he wanted a baby. I was not sure I wanted to be around without the baby. We barely talked during the two and a half hours up to the cottage. I sat curled up in a fetal position in the car, trying to fall asleep in between the sobs.

Brenda finally decided on the aggressive treatment program. It meant that in addition to experiencing total hair loss, nausea and fatigue, she would likely go into early menopause. The first three side effects she could handle, but early menopause was heartbreaking.

🌿 The thought of putting poison in my body that would likely prevent me from ever conceiving was the biggest decision I ever had to make.

The hardest loss of all was not being able to conceive my own child. As a little girl you think of growing up, getting married and getting pregnant. You don't think of problems with fertility or getting cancer in your mid-30s and going into early menopause. I felt that I was robbed of the opportunity to have the child I so desperately wanted.

Brenda's depiction of her dragon captures her panic, her sorrow and her loss.

> 🕊 After lurking around the house, the dragon broke in. It grabbed the most precious thing in the house – and left.
>
> I felt like a mother bird who is watching her baby when a hawk swoops down and rips the baby from the nest. The mother bird circles around but to no avail. The hawk flies away with the tiny bird tight in its grip. All you can see is the panic in the baby bird's eyes and the despair in the mother's eyes.

When Chantal described the world that she had lost to breast cancer, she described a state that had much in common with the world before Grendel.

> 🕊 Once my inner world was a sunny place where the dragon rested peacefully and the flowers bloomed; they were so beautiful with their thousand different colors spread out over miles and miles. The bird song was so joyful, and the sky was so blue with only a few white clouds.... I can see myself just walking around, breathing deeply, with children not far away playing, laughing, and their faces filled with honest and true expression. All was well.

But when the dragon attacked, the sun went out of her world. Gone were the carefree days of her past and her hope for the future. During the "twilight days" that followed her diagnosis, she, like so many other survivors, felt that her life had ended. As Akky said, "Once you get bitten by this dragon, you become part of its world."

In its deadly aspect, the dragon is the ultimate predator. It wipes away past, present and future, leaving in its wake a ruined land, spirits devastated and numb, minds anxious, hearts broken, bodies mutilated. The dragon of breast cancer attacks a woman in the most sensitive place of all – her sexuality, the seat of her identity and feminine power. It is a wound equal in magnitude to that of the mythical Fisher King, who suffered an injury to the groin that caused his country to become a wasteland.

Yet, within the mysterious powers of destruction are the equally mysterious powers of creation. Deep under the ruins of the old life, new seeds begin to stir; sleeping spirits are roused and warriors are born.

III

Facing the Dragon

For 12 years the malevolent dragon holds the country of Denmark hostage, killing at his pleasure. He rules the glittering Hall by night, and King Hrothgar is powerless against him. Then one day a warrior named Beowulf, who lives in a neighboring land, hears about Grendel's marauding. He is an expert dragon slayer, equal to none, and when he learns of the Danish king's problem, he travels to Denmark by boat, accompanied by a troupe of his best warriors. Swift as a seabird he sails, urged on by a favorable wind.

When he arrives at the coast, he introduces himself to the watchman as one who knows how to overcome dragons, and who can offer the King assistance and calm counsel. The watchman is impressed by the warrior, and he leads him and his entourage down a paved road to the King's Hall. When the King sees Beowulf, he greets him warmly, for he remembers meeting him as a child.

THE HEROINE RISES

Like Beowulf, who traveled swiftly over the water to help the King deal with the dragon, a heroic spirit within the survivors rose to the occasion when their lives were deeply challenged. This heroic spirit was present from the very beginning of Akky's journey with cancer.

She had undergone a lumpectomy and the doctor told her that she had a carcinoma of some kind, but not cancer. It was nothing to worry about. *Doesn't carcinoma mean cancer?* Akky wondered. She looked up *carcinoma* in the dictionary and the definition confirmed her suspicion. It was out of character for Akky to question authority, but she bravely followed her own instinct.

> Getting a second opinion was new to me. It took a great deal of courage to ask for something for myself and perhaps offend my doctors.

Later, when she sat in the doctor's office with her husband and heard the doctor recommend a double mastectomy, that same calm spirit of strength presided.

> I was surprised at my relative calmness when the doctor announced I definitely had cancer. I didn't fall apart under the threat of death. I could face it and make decisions without fear.
>
> The diagnosis gave me a lot to think about. Death didn't seem so out of place or unexpected in some ways. I had lived a lifetime and it seemed to be coming to an end.

The "dragon slayer" who emerged to confront the cancer came from a place of deep wisdom, strength and stillness. In fact, for Bernice, the interior guidance was something she associated with another kind of dragon – a wise, benevolent friend.

> He is a gentle creature who lives in the depths of my soul. His proud head supports the grandest gold mustache that glistens, as does each iridescent scale on his body and gilded tail. His eyes are great circles, soft and friendly. He is a jovial fellow with a great smile to match his personality.

The dragon had been with Bernice since childhood. She grew up in the household of an abusive, violent father, and her mother and grandmothers would encourage the children to draw in order to insulate them from what was going on outside. What came out of Bernice's drawings to console her were dragons.

> Whenever I was drawing, my mother knew that I was relaxed, and I remember drawing dragons. They were never ferocious; they were always beautiful – very, very colorful – and their claws weren't really claws, they weren't something to be afraid of.

Bernice's benevolent dragon made an appearance one day when she was 53. She went to get the mail, brought it in and started sorting it into one pile for immediate attention and another for reading at a later date. She came upon a notice reminding her to go for a breast screening.

> Normally I would have put that piece of mail aside and gone on with the household things. I've always put myself on the back burner. But for some reason or another, I do not know, I just had this compelling feeling. I did not put that letter down. I read it, I walked from my living room straight to the telephone and made the appointment. I've never done that before in my life, never ever. And there was a feeling, as soon as I made the appointment of, um, oh, how can I explain it, like when somebody says, "Oh, a job well done!"

Bernice later recognized that "compelling feeling" as her dragon guide and companion, who was like the counselor that Beowulf became to the King.

> "Make the appointment – do not wait!" my dragon encouraged me on the day I received the breast screening message. On that very day we started on our journey together – my dragon and I. He waited patiently for the right moment in time to awaken from his wonderful dreams. He did not strike

out to make himself known to me. Being compassionate, he took his time – uncoiling each section of his magnificent self before nudging me awake too. He knew that I needed to make serious changes. He helped me and I thank him.

FACING THE DRAGON

The survivors met the adversity of cancer with an equally powerful challenger within, who counseled them to stop running, take a stand and meet the dragon eye-to-eye. Franci's moment of reckoning came in the middle of the night when she awoke in terror after a nightmare.

> ❧ I had a very bad dream, being chased by bad guys who were trying to kill me. I was running in a labyrinth, unable to find the exit, trying hard to protect myself. I had been shot several times and was desperately trying to find someone to help me. I did not want to be alone. This was my subconscious obviously telling me something. I bolted up from my sleep at around 3 a.m., perspiring and bawling. I don't think I had cried that hard up to that moment. My family support was diverted because my cousin was dying. I was really alone, I had my own fears, I was frustrated with my feelings and I was scared.
>
> I realized that I had to fight this thing on my own.

Franci expressed what all the women came to in their own way – that she was the only one who could save her. Like Beowulf, she might have a troupe of warriors working on her behalf, but she was the one in charge. When the women claimed the solitary role of commander, their minds became clear. They began to gather intelligence on the opposition, to determine what they were up against. This was a time of reading books, consulting doctors and examining the options.

There were many choices to be made about how to deal with the cancer, hard choices that would affect the rest of their lives. "Should I have chemo and, if so, how much and how strong? Do I have a lumpectomy or a mastectomy, and if I have a mastectomy, do I take the risk of a reconstruction, even though I won't be able to feel a lump should the cancer recur?" For years to come they would wonder over the choices they made, never completely certain they had made the right ones.

Akky chose to have a double mastectomy followed by reconstructive surgery.

> I had to make choices about my treatment. I went for more consultations and read books. I gathered information and people who would support my decisions. It seemed the double mastectomy would give me the best chance of survival, so I went for that, realizing it was my body and I could choose to do what I wanted. If I did survive I wanted to have breasts and so I decided to have a reconstruction using my own tissue. I was going to focus on health and life, on looking and feeling good, and that meant reconstruction. I did not want to be reminded every morning of the double mastectomy. I thought I would look ugly and mutilated.

In addition to making decisions about types of treatment available, the women made decisions about how they were going to live the rest of their lives. They made choices about relationships and values; about who and what was important in their lives; about the attitude they would bring to living and dying. As Cathy said:

> I was faced with the decision of how I wanted to live my life. I felt I had to assess what my priorities were and try to live

each day to the fullest. This sounds clichéd, but I think that until you're faced with such a major life-altering experience, you go through the motions and never triage what's truly important in your life. I made some major choices about how I was going to spend my days. I decided that even though my work was important and valuable, I couldn't keep up the rat-race pace. I reduced my workweek to three days, which allows me now to spend time volunteering, taking care of my household, nurturing my relationships with family and friends, taking care of myself and, of course, paddling my dragon boat. I came to realize how precious time is.

Once they took command, the survivors found that support flowed to them from many sources: family, friends, neighbors, staff at work and even strangers. They felt they were at the helm, pilot of their own craft, like Beowulf sailing through the waters to Denmark.

Confronting Fear

After Beowulf arrives, King Hrothgar gives a feast in his honor. Once again the Hall is brightened by laughter and good cheer, and the heroes swap tales about past adventures. Beowulf says there is nothing more important than courage when dealing with dragons. "Fate will often spare a man if his courage is good," he declares.

As the feast winds down, the King and the Queen go to bed, and the warriors settle in for the night. To the surprise of the armored men, who fully expect to be woken by Grendel, Beowulf removes his iron breast-mail, his helmet and sword. He tells his companions that he does not count himself less in strength than Grendel, and he intends to fight him in hand-to-hand combat. "Unarmed he shall face me," says Beowulf, "if face me he dares."

Beowulf lies down and the tired sea voyagers fall asleep. But the warrior stays awake, waiting for the dragon, kindling within him a fighting fury. When Grendel comes slinking down from the moors, the hero is ready. The dragon gets through the doors easily; though they are bolted with iron bars, he hardly has to touch them and the bolts break free.

The warrior remains motionless and watches every move that the dragon makes. He studies how Grendel attacks, and does not flinch even as the dragon seizes a man, butchers him and devours him in lumps. Then with an open claw Grendel reaches for Beowulf, who lies on the bed. The hero stays his arm and catches the dragon's hand in a death grip. Terrified, the dragon tries to break away, but he cannot. Beowulf stands up, holding on to the dragon with a grip so tight that the monster's fingers begin to split apart. Hearing the noise, Beowulf's men leap to their feet and slash away at the dragon with their swords, but to no avail. They do not know that the dragon has created a spell against weaponry. But Beowulf knows, and he maintains his hold. The dragon's sinews and muscles burst open and at last, fatally wounded, he tears himself away. Leaving his arm in the hero's hand, Grendel makes for the marshes to die.

Marianne Primeau was diagnosed with cancer when she was 39 years old. She had gone through four miscarriages and had finally given birth to a baby girl. Three years later cancer burst into her life and ruined her joy. All the way through chemo and radiation treatments, Marianne felt like the dragon's hostage.

> 🍃 When it is inactive, the dragon sits there blowing just enough smoke to be irritating. And I am not afraid during these times. Then the main fiery blow begins, and I want to run and get away. But there is no escape. I can't outrun it.

My feet are moving in slow motion. The hot, fiery breath scares me. The burn caused is so painful and the healing is so slow. I'm unsettled. I can't sleep at night. I never know how long the blow will last or what damage it will do. I don't know if my body will protect me from the painful burn or if the damaged spot will ever heal.

Marianne went through all the necessary steps to get treatment, but she continued to feel under siege, controlled by this unpredictable, volcanic beast. At first she was furious with God. But as time went by, Marianne came to a realization.

🍃 I didn't want to go to church for a long time after being diagnosed. I felt God had let me down. I felt I was a good person. Why did this happen to me? I'd think of all the unkind people out there and get so angry. In time I came around and came to think God is not the problem. *God didn't give me breast cancer but the strength and courage I need to fight it.*

Marianne's realization transferred the strength from the cancer to herself, and put her on equal ground with the dragon. Instead of directing her fury against God, she put the power of God on her own side and made herself equal in strength to the dragon.

It is worth noting that while waiting for the dragon to enter the room, Beowulf was consciously building a fury within him in preparation for his battle with the beast. In the Indo-European "heroic" vocabulary, words like *furor, ferg, wut, menos* denoted the extreme internal heat that the hero summons before combat. Humans have long known that fueling this inner fire can turn a mere mortal into a superhuman challenger.

Helen Sharpe made herself a warrior from the moment she found out what she was up against. Helen was diagnosed in April 1973, a month before her 41st birthday. Her cancer came as a surprise. She had been preparing for the Passover holiday and was in perfect health, leading a happy and "well-rounded life as a wife, mother, volunteer, part-time university student and performer in amateur musical comedy." Back in the 1970s, when surgeons did a biopsy and found the mass to be cancerous, they went straight on to perform a mastectomy without waking the woman. That's exactly what happened to Helen, but she was not about to give the dragon any ground.

> I woke up, not knowing the outcome. I felt for my breast – it wasn't there.
> I said, "Now I am an *Amazon*."

Dragon stories around the world convey the same message: the way to meet a dragon is to uphold the *conviction* that the dragon – however alarming he appears – is not as strong as his human opponent. For example, in the Chinese tale of "The Dragon King's Daughter," a mortal man named Liu is visiting the underwater palace of the Dragon King when his fearsome brother, the Dragon Lord, comes storming into the hall. Dragging a jade pillar and sporting a flaming mane, this crimson dragon is a thousand feet in length and throws lightning bolts in every direction, followed by thunder, hail and snow. Needless to say, poor Liu is panic-stricken. The Dragon King tells the man not to mind his brother because he is a bit of a show-off. So later, when the Dragon Lord attempts to scare Liu into making a deal with him, the man says to the dragon, "Although I am small enough to hide under one of your scales, I am not afraid of your anger," and his statement wins him the dragon's respect and friendship.

When the survivors stood their ground, when they looked the disease straight in the eye and observed its ways and means, they gathered power over it. Akky described her dragon as a poisonous shape-shifter whose power came from its slippery, secretive nature and the fact that it hid in the darkness formed by everything she had previously ignored or avoided.

    🧬 My dragon was slimy, brown-green and ugly. Fierce and fire-breathing, it lay in its dark and dingy cave waiting for victims to wander by. It waited on top of filth and ugliness and stench, hiding its secrets.

    It could slither into your life without warning, invading every part without you knowing it. It could be solid and seen, or liquid and changing. It could vaporize and show up elsewhere in a different form.

Akky discovered that the dragon's power came from its ability to hide. When she looked right at it without shrinking in fear or horror, she exposed its ways and means.

    🧬 The dragon had gotten me and there was no escape. After I tried denying it, crying about it, hiding from it, being terrorized and frozen by it, the dragon was still there. I could not get rid of it. I could no longer put off dealing with unpleasantness, ugliness, mutilation, horror and even death.

    I could let others try and get rid of it for me while I hid, but it was me it had attacked. I could wait and see if it would go away by itself, but it could and probably would completely devour me. I could not sit around and wait for it to do that. I had to find out what I was dealing with. I had to find out if this dragon was going to kill me or if something could be done. What was a realistic plan?

    First I had to face the beast in the eye and learn all I could about it. It was not easy. At times I simply couldn't read, and then my husband, Henry, read to me. The more I learned, the less frightening and mysterious the dragon became. As I gathered information and talked to people, the dragon became solid and real.

Like Beowulf, Akky examined the way her adversary moved and attacked. When she looked at it with a dispassionate, almost clinical eye, she gained a clear view of what she was up against. She broke the dragon's spell – and it solidified, shrank and ultimately submitted.

Taming the Dragon

The encounter with cancer is a long-term struggle with a dragon who has its victims at its mercy as long as they are afraid. The survivors found that they could regain control and "tame the dragon" if they met fear not as the dragon would expect but with their own unique (and very human) powers of stillness, humor and creativity.

The battle was an extended engagement that required the survivors to maintain their hold on the dragon through surgery, chemotherapy and radiation. Chemotherapy, while it destroys the cancer, also poisons the whole system and undermines the strength of body and mind. Franci described what those hard days – and nights – of treatment were like.

> I didn't know how long chemo was, what it was going to feel like, how I was going to feel after. I was terrified. I had heard that chemo makes you sick, makes you tired. I saw my cousin Susan go through chemo and I saw what it had done to her.
>
> The first time I went, it took them a long time to get the intravenous needles into my hand – six tries. You think, *Is this what it's going to be like every time?* Once they administered the drug I sat there for about an hour. The drug is administered as a drip, so it's not pure drug.
>
> I was scared that I would be sick right away. For the first

session. I brought barf bags with me just in case. You just don't know. I was okay. I went right home, though, and went to sleep. Then, when I woke up, I didn't feel great. It takes a few days for the drugs to go through you. They make you feel like you have a really bad flu. I got the treatment on Thursday and usually by Monday I was feeling better. I would spend the weekends lying low. I read. If I could go out, I would. I kept myself busy. I went to the movies. I tried to go to the gym. People would come by and see me during the day, but the nights were bad.

At night I would lie in bed with tears rolling down the side of my face, telling myself, *You will be fine – you will get through this!* I was nauseous from the poison they injected into my body during the day. (You know that feeling when all you want to do is throw up to feel better, but you can't?) I was alone. There was no one to hold or cuddle me, no one to kiss me good night. Closing my eyes, I would feel the heavy tiredness and tension in my body. I would try to relax. I kept fighting those inner dark thoughts and feelings, the what-ifs, as I sank into sleep. Then the dreams began. Total anxiety.... They were quite vivid, such as getting shot but not dying; lying there feeling the pain from the bullets, trying to keep moving. Caught in a maze while being chased, not able to find the exit; stuck in an elevator on my way to chemo and no one able to find me....I woke from these horrific dreams shaking, crying, perspiring and scared.

I had 12 treatments, two weeks a month for six months, followed by radiation. The radiation affects you internally, and then it comes to the surface. They tell you it's going to be like a bad sunburn. You think, *Oh, I can handle that*, but inside where I was radiated, it is still so tender. Under my arm at the site of my surgical incision, my skin was split wide open, really badly burned. And under my breast it was raw – *raw.*

Radiation burned the crap out of me, from the inside out. When you put something in a microwave, it cooks from the inside out. That's exactly what it's like. Still, compared to chemo, radiation is a walk in the park.

Franci dealt with chemo and radiation by maintaining as normal a routine as possible. As she described in her dragon imagery, all the way through the dragon's fiery blow, she kept on moving. "I could feel myself consumed by the burning flame, but I did not stop moving," she wrote. Every day she would make a point of having a shower, getting dressed, putting on makeup and going out for a walk. She told herself that if she looked okay, she was okay. On a moment-to-moment basis she asserted her warrior spirit – but the poison and the burn were not something she would soon forget.

The weakening effect of chemotherapy and the need to keep order in the household nearly overwhelmed some women. Julie Dubuc, who is a visual artist living in Winnipeg, is also a mother of five children ranging from 4 to 22 years of age. She was in her mid-40s when her cancer was found, shortly after the birth of her last child. It had spread to one lymph node. Her oncologist advised her to have chemotherapy followed by 25 radiation treatments. Julie wasn't sure she wanted to go through with the chemotherapy. She had many loved ones who needed her, and her partner, Denis, had epilepsy. Chemo would prove to be a bumpy ride.

🖋 The night after my first treatment, I was feeling quite nauseous and needed to sleep. Denis had three grand mal seizures that night. Seizures are sometimes brought on by stress and he is very sensitive. Grand mal seizures are not pleasant to witness, which added to my nausea. Worse, though, is the fact that following a seizure, never mind three, the patient is then unconscious for the next 12 to 24 hours.

Denis had had a very hard night and slept the entire 24 hours following. I had to get up in the morning to care for our daughter as well as try to help Denis as much as I could. It was a difficult couple of days. In the 21 days that followed I had decided several times to quit my chemo treatments, and each time I changed my mind again. I went for my second treatment still not knowing what I should do. The same thing occurred the night of my second treatment: Denis again had three grand mal seizures and, again, was incapacitated the following day. This time I was in pretty rough shape and found it very difficult to manage. My older children except one were living with their dad at the time and I did not have them around to help. I was very depressed, tired, and I felt like I was drowning. The stress was overwhelming.

My third treatment was scheduled on December 16, but due to a low blood count it was postponed a week. I refused to take the treatment on the 23rd, as I wanted to be able to cook Christmas dinner for my children. It was postponed until after the new year.

During the week before Christmas, Denis suffered a hysterical seizure, which lasted about one week. He was not able to sleep and suffered hallucinations as well as giddiness and depression. I was so stressed out by this and trying to get ready for Christmas with my children that I did not feel that I could handle anything else.

It was Julie's creative power as an artist that enabled her to stay in charge. An idea for a painting came to her in the middle of the night.

🍃 I knew that I was strong enough to handle the drugs, but I did not know if I could manage chemo and deal with the stresses of my home life. One night about three a.m., not being able to sleep, worrying about these life-threatening decisions that I was forced to make, I suddenly had an image. I saw myself as a very fragile bubble floating down this long misty tunnel of life, and having to steer past broken shards of glass that emerged out of the mist. I painted the image and called it *Living on the Edge*. The painting helped me to accept my circumstances and make the best of the situation. I did quit my treatments for seven weeks but eventually went back and completed seven chemotherapy sessions.

When Julie saw her predicament in the form of an image, she understood the challenge ahead and what was required of her. She conquered her fears and gained power over the dragon by transforming the ordeal into a creative project that inspired and excited her. It gave her the ability to keep an even keel over the days and nights of the battle.

🖋 There is an interesting thing that happens when I paint... the painted image becomes my reality. I can change my reality by changing the image. It's magic in a way. It is a way to keep me grounded. Doing something of value keeps me connected to a normal life. When I am painting, I feel normal.

Cathy was weakened from the moment she learned the news of her cancer. She had never been undermined to such a degree by anything in her life.

🖋 Initially the dragon stripped me of my strength. I had never felt so weak as the day when I was diagnosed. My initial reaction wouldn't allow me to think long-term at all. I didn't think I would live through the week, never mind see old age. I had my first chemotherapy treatment on December 24, 1996. *Merry Christmas.* The next day I received a roll of 250 return address labels from Santa in my stocking. I remember looking at them thinking, *I will never have a chance to use up all of the labels before I die.*

Yet Cathy would not allow herself to succumb to weakness. From the beginning she put herself in charge of rebuilding her self-confidence. Lapses into weakness would occur from time to time, but she allowed them to occur only for brief moments. Cathy met her adversary with humor and an absolute resolve not to let it gain the upper hand. Every setback made her stronger – but it was no joyride. She called the process of taming her dragon a "bronco-busting event."

> That dragon didn't want to be ridden and quite frankly I had never dreamed of being a cowgirl. There was definitely a power struggle between the dragon and me as I fought with how I was going to overcome this burden that I was faced with. Initially, when I was at my weakest, the dragon was bucking pretty good. But from the moment I had my first treatment planning session with the surgeon, I was in control. We had an action plan and we were moving forward. For the first while I needed training wheels for my dragon, and there were certainly some setbacks as I learned to retake control of the reins. But the dragon was never able to throw me off. What made it possible for me to stay on·for the ride was my instinct to survive. I don't think that it was ever a conscious choice that I made, just something that I knew I had to do. I am still riding the dragon today; however, our scene of bronco-busting is now closer to that of elegant show jumping. I am in control of the reins.

The survivors found that they could put the dragon at a disadvantage by not acting out of fear. When they asserted themselves, the dragon became more manageable, and the "dragon slayer" made contact with a source of supreme strength. As Cathy said:

> I believe now that I have greater ferocity than before, with a strength that is more directed and easier to draw on. I am much more assertive. I have developed a "take charge" attitude in my life. I try not to let things just happen to me. I control and take an active role in shaping my destiny. I also gained a certain veracity. By that I mean that I am more truthful with myself. So, in the long run I think I can say that I gained more from that dragon than it took away from me. NA, NA, NA, NA, NA!

Like Cathy, Helen tamed her dragon with humor and Amazonian courage. From the moment she lost her breast, she claimed the loss as the mark of a warrior's achievement and turned it into an opportunity for amusement.

> I was still me. This dragon took nothing intrinsic from me, only a body part, the lack of which I learned to accept quickly, and which became and continues to be a source of amusement to all who know me. My "boob" has floated up out of my bathing suit and bobbed on the surface of a crowded swimming pool, fallen to the floor at a party during an unfortunate dance move and has been left behind in more than one hotel!

The idea of "taming the dragon" is an old one that can be found in ancient Chinese books. According to these accounts, tamed dragons once pulled the chariots of legendary kings, and one family was even purported to breed tamed dragons for the emperors. In *Dragons and Dragon Lore*, Ernest Ingersoll writes that "it later became the custom to ornament the prows of pleasure-junks with dragon heads, and certain kinds of long, slender boats are known as 'dragon-boats' to this day." And Ingersoll notes that in the *Book of Changes* the symbolism of the dragon was intricately woven with royal and heroic acts. Those who ascended to the "dragon-throne" were said to be persons with a high degree of self-control and powers that verged on the supernatural.

Allies

Once the survivors took charge and set a course for recovery, their families, loved ones and even strangers supported them in many wonderful ways. After her surgery, Karen Kellner came home with a renewed purpose to live a healthy life, and her family followed her direction.

> ◖ The day after I came home I took my family up to our local health food store and spent a ton of money – cookbooks and food items so foreign to me (at the time) my kids were making gross sounds. I laugh at it now, but at the time I was out to rescue my life.

Karen also learned to accept help from allies in a way she never had before.

> ◖ When my neighbors offered to help with things I said yes. Before diagnosis I was "superwoman." I could do everything! Accepting a helping hand from friends let alone neighbors was not within my range of capacity. Reaching out was really hard.

Support often came from surprising places, as Akky discovered when she pursued the idea of having reconstructive surgery. She came into the kitchen one day to see her son poring over books that would normally not be admitted there.

> ◖ My middle son Jonathan found some books on reconstruction and commented how all the women looked better after their reconstruction. I saw him leafing through books with

pictures of topless women and wondered how he could be doing such a thing right under my nose on the kitchen table. He helped me to feel I would look fine to him no matter what I chose to do.

Marianne too was surprised by the support she received from her child. During her treatment she had been putting on a brave face and trying to maintain a sense of normalcy in the household so that her three-year-old daughter would remain secure and happy. But then one day her daughter demonstrated a remarkable empathy.

> I was playing on the bed with my daughter. My wig slipped a bit and I quickly tugged it back on. But she caught me. She realized it was a wig. She pulled the wig off and rubbed my bald head with her tiny gentle hand, and she said, "I'm so sorry this happened to you." The tears fell and we hugged.

Wherever they came from, the allies who supported the survivors in their battle with the dragon were dearly remembered for all their own brave deeds and heartfelt gestures. And as Cathy pointed out, they provided a valuable lesson in "how to be a friend, sister and partner."

> I was very fortunate to have supportive people around me throughout this ordeal. I had some very dear friends who really stepped up to help me, just by letting me know that they were there. There wasn't a day that went by that one of them wasn't checking in to see if I needed anything. My family members, however, were the most important to me at this time. My sisters called or stopped by daily, sometimes several times, to check on me, see what I was up to, and just to chat. I valued those visits and phone calls immensely, and although we generally talked about "nothing," there was always an undertone of concern for me in their voices.

My husband, Marc, was perhaps the one whom I relied on the most, especially when it felt like the bottom would fall out. I think he was probably the only one who I let see the real fear and hurt that I was experiencing. I didn't want to worry my family and friends. I didn't want them to think that I couldn't cope.

One other person whom I relied on heavily throughout my treatment was J.R. Ewing. Reruns of *Dallas* began simultaneously with my treatments. Every day, no matter what, I stopped what I was doing in order to watch my show. Everyone knew not to call between 10 a.m. and 11 a.m. It was a perfect escape.

One of the most disconcerting features of the dragon is its metamorphic nature. Dragons are not solid creatures; they are fluid, elusive and capable of self-transformation. They are renowned for making themselves dark and invisible or luminous and splendid. They can shrink to the size of a silkworm or swell till they fill the space of heaven and earth. They can move through any barrier or element – air, water or earth.

The elusive, secretive and deadly nature of cancer terrified the survivors. As long as they were controlled by that terror, they were diminished and overwhelmed. But when they stood their ground, they found that the dragon solidified and became a definable, manageable adversary. As the story of *Beowulf* indicates, weaponry is useless in our first meeting with the dragon. The only way to break the dragon's spell is for the dragon slayer to believe in the power of his or her own spirit. Brenda Tierney summed up the attitude when she declared, "I *am* the dragon!" The warrior must be willing to confront the beast, expose it and come to grips with it. Only then will the monster succumb.

IV

In Pursuit of the Dragon

After Beowulf defeats Grendel with the power of his own grip, the fatally wounded dragon staggers back to his joyless lair. Beowulf and warriors follow the bloody dragon tracks and finish him off there. But that isn't the end of the story. Furious over the death of her son, Grendel's mother rises up from the black depths of her home in a deep, cold lake. She is an even more terrible adversary than her son, and after the warriors finish celebrating their victory, she has her revenge. She gets into the Hall at night, grabs the most beloved and well known of all the King's men, and quickly makes off with her trophy. When the tragedy is discovered the next day, Beowulf vows to pursue and destroy her. This time he suits himself up in the finest armor, and he and the King, along with their best warriors, set forth into the land of the dragon – a little-known country of craggy peaks, wolf-slopes, windswept headlands, perilous paths and boggy moors.

Going into the Unknown

Once the survivors rose to meet the challenge of their cancer, they had to go in active pursuit of their lives, chasing the dragon down to recover what they had lost. The road ahead led through wild, unfamiliar regions, marked by mists, chasms and lonely, difficult crossings. Looking back on the road that she had traveled from diagnosis through to recovery, Julie Dubuc said:

> ❧ Imagine that you are standing high up on the edge of a cliff, and in order to continue on your journey you are faced with having to cross the canyon on a very old and rickety suspension bridge. Then you have to crawl along a narrow ledge and slowly descend along the edge of the cliff. The path continues through a very dense and dark misty fog and crosses the canyon in the form of a narrow ledge high up in the air with only the mist to comfort and caress you. The world of the normal, the realm that you desperately would like to return to, is on the other side of the canyon and you can just barely make it out in the far distance. This is where I was as I faced surgery, chemo and radiation. It can be a very dangerous and scary journey. The best comfort I can offer is to say, "It's just one step at a time. Put one foot in front of the other and you'll eventually get there."

After diagnosis, "life became an emergency," as Pamela Robbins said. There was no time to procrastinate or worry over trivial matters. Many of the survivors noted, "I stopped sweating the small stuff." As they began to pursue their health and their dreams, they headed into the unknown – a region long associated with dragons. As old maps indicate, cartographers marked the areas that had not been explored or charted with the symbol of the dragon.

Once she had recovered from the initial shock of her diagnosis, Akky and her husband, Henry, quite literally went into the unknown. Akky had four weeks to wait before her surgery and she couldn't imagine how she would survive the eight-hour operation ahead. Then the opportunity to go to the Arctic came up and Akky wanted to go. Henry wasn't sure that they could afford the trip, but Akky insisted, saying, "I can't afford *not* to."

She wanted to do some living if she was going to die. So she and Henry set off on a hiking and canoeing trip to a region called Mesa Incognita, a barren territory in Baffin Island, not unlike the one described in *Beowulf*.

> It was a mountainous landscape with rounded, glaciated hills, 3,000 feet high. The hills supported very little vegetation, only lichen, mosses and very low willows creeping on the ground in sheltered areas. We crossed through bogs, puddles, rivers and waterfalls. The mist rising in places was like the breath of dragons, and we worried about polar bears who were all around us, and caribou who might trample our campsite. We went in July, the warmest season, but even then it was very rainy, foggy and cold; the most chilling damp imaginable. A few degrees cooler and it would have been snowing. There were some sunny days, and when we were walking, we would have to take off layers but then bundle up again the minute we stopped. It got dusky at night, but by two o'clock in the morning the light was back.

On the island, Akky and her husband stayed with an Inuit family who exposed them to a timeless world completely beyond the scope of their experience, where the people still hunted seal, polar bear and fox, as their ancestors had done – and Akky had the kind of adventure she had been missing all her life.

Akky's venture into Mesa Incognita expressed the attitude that many women assumed after they came to terms with their diagnosis. Like the classic warriors and dragon slayers before them, they went forth bravely into uncharted territory, pursuing their dreams with uncommon vigor. For this engagement with the dragon, they needed to arm themselves with all the weaponry they had at their disposal – knowledge, technology and troops. Marian expressed how to prepare for battle:

❧ Arm yourself and face the dragon squarely. Arm yourself with humor, because it gives you distance and perspective in the course of battle. Arm yourself with knowledge, because it will help you learn how to fight the dragon. Arm yourself with the minutiae of daily life, because it reminds you that the world is still there and that you are a part of it. Arm yourself with friends and loved ones, because they provide hope and strength in your darkest hours.

PURSUING THE DRAGON

All the survivors had a ferocious determination to pursue their health to whatever limit they were taken. Some faced nearly impossible odds, and yet they would not acquiesce. Evelyn, whose ordeal began when she slipped on the carpet, was given 18 months to live. Her oncologist offered her standard chemotherapy until the disease progressed, but that was all the medical system could offer her. It seemed inevitable that she would die. But Evelyn was a fighter, and it wasn't long before she found another way.

❧ I watched a program on television about a new experimental treatment that they seemed to be having great success with in Sudbury called stem cell transplants.

In a stem cell transplant, the stem cells (immature blood cells – neither white nor red) are collected after you are given high-dose chemotherapy. Then they reinfuse you with the collected stem cells. If they reinfuse you with diseased stem cells, they are giving you back cancer cells.

I asked my oncologist about it, but he was reluctant to help, so I made an appointment myself, and off I went to Sudbury.

In Sudbury, Evelyn was told that she did not fit their protocol, which was disappointing, but they did give her some hope. In three months' time they would be conducting another clinical trial and they suggested that she might meet those criteria. They advised her to wait and reconnect with them in three months.

    🌿 Three months stretched to six months, at which time they asked me to have a bone marrow aspiration before entering into their clinical trial. The procedure showed that the cancer had advanced into my bone marrow, which automatically disqualified me from the clinical trial. There was nothing else they could do.

Until that moment Evelyn had hoped she would find a way to live, but she came away from Sudbury heartbroken.

    🌿 I had been my own advocate, and I had worked so hard and waited so patiently for the right protocol, only to be turned away in the end because the cancer had advanced into my bone marrow. I think the doctors in Sudbury probably did as much as most doctors could when they tell you such devastating news, but it never seems like enough to me – it's so clinical, so cut and dried. When I think about it now, I don't know what they could have done differently, but it seems to me that in some ways they have not come very far, at least from an emotional point of view. It was a devastating four-and-a-half-hour drive home from Sudbury with my husband, my mother, a friend and my nine-year-old daughter. I don't think one of us spoke a word.

Even so, Evelyn kept fighting. She followed up on the doctors in the U.S. who were doing stem cell transplants with purging. (Purging means that the tumor cells are removed and destroyed before transplantation.) She was able to track down a doctor in Denver,

Colorado, who agreed to see her. So Evelyn and her husband prepared to fly to the United States.

🌿 I had a nine-year-old daughter to raise, a husband who needed me and, damn it, I wanted to live. I had been tenacious my whole life, and I wasn't about to change.

As we will see later, Evelyn would not give up her battle for life, wherever it took her. And she wasn't alone. Brenda Welsh also went in hot pursuit of the dragon who took her dream baby, and her determination to win her dream back from the dragon only fueled her campaign for health.

🌿 I would chase that dragon with every bit of my strength to make it retreat. It had a part of my flesh and my little innocent dream tucked tightly under its massive arm, and I knew I could not free the dream without causing my own death. It stole my dream to conceive a child, but I refused to let the dragon feel a sense of victory.

I think that all along I had the dragon by the tail. I refused to let go. I kept slowly climbing up the back of the dragon. Several times I fell, but I just dusted myself off and tried again. I kept battling using different techniques, trying different ways to fight back. I refused to give up.

In November 1997, Brenda stopped menstruating – and gone was the hope of having her own child. However, she soon found a new pathway and began to explore surrogacy. It proved to be a complicated and risky proposition, but Brenda pursued the possibility anyway.

🌿 In Canada, the person carrying the baby cannot give the egg, so in actual fact I needed two women to assist me. I registered for the egg donation program because I thought that it would be too difficult psychologically for my sister to give her eggs. I was also concerned that she would have to take hormones to make multiple eggs. I was fearful that it could cause her to get breast cancer. If for some reason she had a trace of breast cancer in her system and the procedure caused it to spread, I could never forgive myself. I was not prepared to take any chances. For several months I contemplated the possibility of surrogacy. My sister, my sister-in-law and a friend all offered to assist us. I was humbled by their kindness.

Eventually Brenda gave up the surrogacy option because of the ramifications and the risks. But pursuing surrogacy had served a purpose. It had given her the hope that had sustained her through six months of aggressive chemotherapy. In the end, she let go of the surrogacy option, but her pursuit continued. She and Stephen began looking into adoption.

In April 1997 we attended our first adoption meeting, and we learned about our options. A women spoke about her experience adopting a little girl from China. Her little girl's name was Jemma. As I heard her story I started to feel very drawn to the possibility of adopting a little girl from China.

With private adoptions the couples basically had to find their own expecting mother. Couples were actually making up business cards and handing them out at parties and sending letters to doctors trying to find a woman who was interested in giving up her child.

As I was working for the Children's Aid Society of Toronto, I thought that it might be easier to just adopt through my place of employment. Then I found out that for confidentiality reasons I would have to have the home study done by another organization. My husband and I went to an information session at the Catholic Children's Aid Society. We felt discouraged by the waiting period and disappointed that they

were concerned about my diagnosis. We learned how difficult it was to get a child under one year old. They also asked
us if we were willing to accept a special needs child. We
decided not to proceed.

Of the new options, one avenue in particular attracted Brenda
and she couldn't get it out of her mind.

     ❦ I kept thinking of this little girl from China and how little
girls were not valued as much as boys. In the summer of 1997
we attended our first meeting with Open Arms, an adoption
agency. After meeting the facilitator's daughter, who was
adopted from China, and after seeing their video, I just knew
that adopting from China was my destiny. I felt at peace with
myself when I thought about the possibility of adopting a
baby from an orphanage in China. It was comforting to think
that I would give a child a chance in life who otherwise might
never be truly loved by someone.

Brenda completed her chemotherapy and radiation, and went
forward with her new adoption plans, but then, to her shock, she
rammed up against what seemed like an insurmountable obstacle.

     ❦ In the summer of 1997 we found a social worker and started
the process. But then we were told that because I had a life-
threatening illness, it was unlikely that I would be approved.
I remember feeling devastated and angry. I was a good person.
I had 15 wonderful nieces and nephews and a family so willing
to share their love with another child. I was university-
educated and had the means to care for a child. I had cancer,
but it was gone.

     I was not dying. I felt that I had so much to offer a child
and I so desperately wanted to have one. I worked as a social
worker for the Children's Aid Society, which was ironic as I

was apprehending children from their parents and now I was being seen as unfit to care for a child. I could not believe I was being turned down. Natural parents were given every opportunity to care for their children. Single men and women were given the opportunity to adopt. It was unfair that I was denied this opportunity. I felt angry and questioned what I had done to deserve this.

Still, Brenda held on to the dragon's tail.

〰 Knowing what I was up against, I had to decide if I would pursue my goal. The next summer – 1998 – I found another social worker who agreed to send a preliminary letter to the Ministry [of Community and Social Services] to get an approval to start the home study. I had to provide my medical history. They did not want to know anything else. I wanted them to know all the good things in my life, but they were only interested in my diagnosis of cancer. It was like that was all that mattered. They could not see beyond the cancer. I ended the letter by saying, "No one can guarantee they will stay healthy. I can only say that I feel great and we plan to live a long, happy life. We give our solemn promise that whatever happens in our lives, our child will be raised in a loving and nurturing environment."

I was turned down.

I was sitting at my desk when I got the call that the Ministry wanted me to be five years cancer-free prior to applying. I was seen as too high-risk. They were worried that I could die and did not want to take that chance. I had already been waiting since 1993 to start my family. I certainly was not prepared to wait until 2002 to start this process.

In the summer of 1999 I started fighting back even harder. I got several letters of support from my doctors, and the

Breast Cancer Foundation wrote a letter of support saying, "The Canadian Breast Cancer Foundation supports the belief that no woman who has battled back from breast cancer should be discriminated against, and therefore we reiterate our support of Brenda and Stephen being afforded the opportunity to share their life and love with an adopted child."

Brenda kept on pursuing her dream long after she had fought back the cancer. Trying to pry her dream baby out of the dragon's clutches would become the struggle of her life, but Brenda kept at it with a tenacity equal to that of the worthiest dragon slayer. She did not know whether she would win the battle, but, as every true warrior knows, the pursuit is everything. As Brenda said:

> ❦ Only a small group of people can live to tell their story of wrestling with a dragon. I walked away wounded but a stronger person for having the courage to fight such a fierce beast.

Winning Life Back

When Anita was first introduced to dragon boating, her response was unexpected and emotional.

> ❦ I was at a breakfast meeting for the Heart and Stroke Foundation in early November of 1999 when the moderator announced the name of a local woman who was trying to start up a dragon boat team in Prince George! I burst into spontaneous tears and everyone at my table agreed that it must be important to me. How right they were!

Every woman had a story about how she first encountered dragon boating and how she instinctively responded to the dragon's call.

Franci was recuperating from surgery when she saw a special on television.

> ❧ I had just had my surgery in October of 1997 (breast cancer awareness month – how ironic). CBC did a special called "Abreast in a Boat" – also the name of the Vancouver dragon boat breast cancer survivor team. I knew of the sport of dragon boating and now became aware of this very special team. The show was empowering. My mother, who is also a breast cancer survivor, was watching the special with me. These women have bonded together and exude such strength and determination as they paddle in their boat. They had overcome something that I was just starting to go through. We wept together watching this, and my mother's exact words to me were: "That will be *you*, Franci. I can just see it! Just give yourself some time...."
>
> From that point on, as I was going through my healing journey, I kept telling people, "I want to dragon boat!" I wanted to be a part of that *spirit of aliveness*!

It is no wonder that so many breast cancer survivors are passionate about dragon boating. Their fight for life has given them a furious will to live and a deep strength. When they see other women racing in the water, their faces strained with the determination to win – they see themselves winning against the dragon.

Their attraction to dragon boating goes right to the roots of the sport. Dragon boating began in ancient China as a means by which to rouse the sky dragons and get them to fight. When the dragons fought in the sky, their breath formed the darkening clouds, their roar made the thunder, and their fire, the lightning. The great storm that followed brought down the life-giving rain. The people would go out on the water in the spring, when the fields were barren and the spirit of the rice seeds had weakened.

With all their might the dragon boaters would race down the river towards the fields, rousing the life forces, energizing the seeds, and defeating the dark shadows of drought, death and disease.

Like the rice seeds themselves, the women started dragon boating when they were feeling weakened by chemotherapy and surgery. Their coaches taught them to fight back the weakness, to dig deep for strength. As Evelyn said:

> One evening while the team was out on Lake Ontario practicing, one of the coaches began referring to the women in the boat as "dragon slayers" who were going to conquer the dragon, and he said, "Think of the water as the cancer, and when your paddle hits that water think of it as a fight, the fight of your life, and that you are slaying the dragon."

For breast cancer survivors, every race is a ritual battle with the dragon. They call it "winning against Lane 11." While 10 boats line up to race, they imagine Lane 11 to be occupied by the dragon of cancer. The women may appear to be racing against each other, but they are really racing against cancer, winning their lives back from the dragon. With every stroke they recover the strength and the life that the dragon has taken from them. Said Cathy:

> From the depth of my lowest point I made the decision to fight back. I wasn't going to let this thing control me or take over my life. I developed a serious "kick-butt" attitude. I was going to fight this with every weapon that the medical community had to offer. I would not lose.
>
> I get chills when I think about getting into the boat to race, or even to practice, for that matter. When I enter that boat I take on a persona that doesn't appear in my everyday life. I become somewhat ruthless and aggressive in my attempt to win the race. I push myself to the limit, all to show this breast

cancer dragon that it can't push me or my friends around. It really gives me a sense of control over my life.

Pulling to the limits of her strength, each woman is winning something back from the dragon. For Kaethe Lawn of Victoria, B.C., the loss was trust. Kaethe was diagnosed in her 40s, and up until that time she had assumed her body would be there for her.

> Cancer was a profoundly sobering experience, a letting go of what until then had supported me in my life's struggles. I could no longer trust my body to respond appropriately. Even though I did the right things, I could still suddenly become very ill, for no apparent reason.
>
> This shook me deeply, and to this day I feel a sense of betrayal.

In every race, Kaethe restores the connection between mind and body that was severed through the experience of cancer, slowly repairing her trust in the capacity of her body to respond to her mind.

> I often approach the limits of my capability. I think this is because of my age (most of my fellow paddlers are younger than I am) and also probably because I am just not very athletic. I have to push myself very hard to be as good as the rest of the team, and that is difficult and often painful for me. I deal with this problem by talking to myself inside. I encourage myself and I do not allow myself to give in. My mind overrides my body and then I can paddle as well as the other women.

Slaying the dragon in a race is a thrill that can hardly be described. It recalls every woman's personal battle with cancer, and she relives it through the ritual of each race. Bernice, who is on the Winnipeg team Chemo Savvy, gave us a picture of what it felt like to be a survivor paddling in a dragon boat race.

🍃 "Paddles up!" There's our cue. Instantly, 20 paddles are extended – to hover just above the choppy water. We are ready. One sharp blast of the horn startles us into action. We stretch out and reach as far as possible into the splashing waves ahead, plunging our paddles as deep as we can.

"Hope! Hope! Hope!" we chant, as our drummer pounds on the huge black drum. She keeps us paddling as one. Whatever we lack in strength, we make up for with our synchronization. We glide over the murky water as if on wings.

The air is packed with excitement. As we approach the midpoint, the crowd is yelling, "Go girls, go!" We pull that much faster – we stretch that much farther – we go all out! My arms are burning. Every part of my body is wound tight like a rubber band, ready to snap into action with our next move.

"Dig!" shouts our steersperson. We now know that we must be neck-and-neck with one or both of the other boats. We heed her command, and with every stroke our 40-foot craft glides forward. "Dig deeper!" she cries out again, so we do.

To keep in sync with my partners, I start to call out, "Dig! Dig deep!" Then someone else takes up the chant, "Dig deep!" With every beat of the drum, each paddle is filled and we recite the words, "Hope! Hope! Hope!"

Our paddles dig deeper and faster. The spectators are shouting louder than before, "Go girls, go!" We're on a high – we push every ounce of weight behind each pull and go like the wind. My surgery side is stinging and my arm is in a knot, but I won't let my "sisters" down. I must keep paddling.

From vocal cords already strained comes the final sign we've been waiting for. "Dig deep! Keep going! You're doing great! Keep going – we're almost there! Dig! Dig deep! Dig deeper!" We paddle as fast as our aching muscles allow.

Thousands of spectators are screaming, "Go Chemo Savvy – Go Chemo Savvy!" Their encouragement gives us that last surge of energy and we push our vessel over the finish line.

We should relax then but cannot. We each toss a pink rose onto the water in memory of the women who lost the hardest race of their lives – then we reach out to each other and cry tears of joy and pride.

Warding off disease and ultimately slaying the dragon of breast cancer is the personal and collective campaign of all the dragon boating survivors. They race to raise funds for breast cancer research, and they race to show others that there is life after breast cancer. As Brenda Tierney said:

> When we paddle in the festival, I know there are women watching us who have had cancer and are looking for a new pathway for themselves. They will be with us next year and will share in the wonderful camaraderie that we experience. They will also have a floating support group to help them through their difficult times.

Many of the survivors' families were also very moved to see their loved ones reasserting themselves in the dragon boat race. Dragon boating expresses to the families and to the crowd that the women – mothers, daughters and sisters – have emerged from their cancer with more energy and hope than ever before. Fran was taken aback by how much pride her family took in her dragon boating.

> One of the by-products of dragon boating was the extreme pride that my family felt. They came and watched me race, and my son took beautiful photographs. I was very touched that my kids would come out and cheer me on. I thought, *I do what I do, and you've got your own lives!* Later, when I came

to the cottage at the lake, I was surprised to find a picture of our team on the fridge with a circle drawn around me and the expression, "Yea Mom!" from my daughter-in-law. That my dragon boating meant so much to them was surprising. I felt that I wasn't being a burden to them any more, and maybe they felt a little freed of worrying about their mother. We had all emerged from the crisis together!

In the spring, when the dragon boats are first brought out of storage, they are blessed and cleansed by Taoist priests. One of the spells that an exorcist from the Chinese province of Hunan casts over the boats is: "As the dark waters down the river flow, so may all maladies, diseases, plagues and death go."

Even today, many Chinese believe that the dragon boat festival falls on one of the unluckiest days of the year. On the fifth day of the fifth month, the forces of life and death are at the height of their conflict; evil is on the loose and demons are everywhere. It is essential to rally the powers of life, guarding oneself and others from reversals of fortune.

For many, the battle to win back life is the most important aspect of dragon boating. The paddlers share the same defiant position: "I'm not going to let this cancer beat me!" From that source of combined power, they draw the strength that they need to slay their dragons. Each tempers her own sword in the fires of the group spirit – winning back the power she has lost and arming herself for the battles ahead.

V

Dark Night, Near Death

Beowulf and his warriors follow the tracks of Grendel's mother into the dark woods, only to find that she lives deep under the gory waters of an inland lake. To slay her, Beowulf has to go into the watery depths of the emotional domain. For this battle he needs all the protection and weaponry he can get. He covers his head with a helmet, his body with a war-corselet so he might not wound his heart, and he seizes a powerful sword. No sooner has he entered the water than the mother of dragons grabs him and dives to the bottom of the lake. They come into a vaulted chamber, and there the battle begins in earnest. Beowulf soon finds that his sword is no use to him against the hideous dragon. It breaks. He stumbles and falls. The dragon sits on his chest and is about to finish him off when suddenly he spies an invincible sword, wrought by giants, lying within reach. He grasps the sword by the hilt, and in one swoop he beheads the dragon.

Meanwhile, on shore, the warriors stare into the gory waters of the lake, heartsick. They have nearly given up hope when, to their amazement, Beowulf rises from the bloody waters – victorious.

SALVATION AT THE BRINK

Beowulf was taken to the brink of death; and while he survived, the poet Qu Yuan did not. Overwhelmed by despair, the poet clasped a

stone to his breast and drowned himself in the river. In their struggle with cancer, many women were taken to that same brink, and
they related deeply and powerfully to the tragedy of Qu Yuan. They
all knew how close one can get to the edge. Julie Dubuc's struggle
with chemotherapy and her husband's epilepsy pushed her to the
very limit of her endurance. She could see how easy it would have
been to succumb, how just a little shove from fate might have sent
her over the side.

> ✺ Probably my darkest hour was a three-day stretch after my
> fourth chemo treatment, when I developed an allergic reac-
> tion either to the drugs or to something that my immune sys-
> tem could not fight off because it was so depleted. I developed
> an entire-body rash in the form of welts. I was so itchy that I
> could not think about anything else. Sleep was out of the ques-
> tion and I stayed up all night applying towels soaked in ice
> water to my body. As I applied the towels, the rash would
> recede but reappear moments later on another area of my
> skin. I was so tired and I felt so defeated. I did not have the
> energy to keep on fighting and felt very alone. I had been
> advised to take Benadryl, but after I took it for two days the
> rash just got worse. I was crying on the phone to my oncologist
> at 7:00 the next morning. The only thing that got me through
> that time was to believe that the drug would work.
>
> Finally, I was prescribed steroids, and within a day or so the
> rash began to recede. It was an agonizing three days and made
> me realize that there does come a point in time when you
> give up and wish to die. If it had gone on much longer, I
> would have reached that point.

Chantal remembers the time when she nearly gave up. She had
taken the giant step of confronting her boyfriend, and she and her
son had moved out. They had gone to live with Chantal's brother,

but it was there that her misery caught up with her. Overwhelmed by the losses of her breast and her hair, and cruelly rejected by her partner, Chantal sank into a deep depression.

🌿 I let myself go, not putting on makeup, staying in my pajamas, not wearing a bra with a prosthesis, wearing a cap instead of a wig – looking sick.

Unexpectedly, her younger brother Alain offered her an opportunity for salvation.

🌿 My brother was about to go out for a beer with his friends. I was ready to stay home, all quiet, feeling depressed. My brother got upset at me. He told me I was letting myself go. I was no longer taking care of my appearance, and I was making sure I looked ugly with my bald head, my pale skin and lack of vitality in my eyes. He "ordered" me to get a grip and to put on makeup, dress up, make my bed and start being active.

My brother's friends convinced me to come along with them. I agreed. I was going to wear my wig, but Alain's friend Stéphane said: "Don't put anything on your head. Come like this, no cap, no scarf and no wig." I started to laugh and felt nervous. I thought he was crazy! But then, he was a true master of conviction. I took a shower, put on my leather pants, my bra with a temporary prosthesis (so what, it did the job!), a nice knitted camisole and my leather "rocker" jacket. Makeup, perfume, jewelry, little booties. A naked head. *Let's go!*

I actually looked great! And I had fun doing it! Feeling the wind on my naked head was a sensual feeling. We went on St-Denis Street in Montreal, in a place called St-Sulpice. It is a famous place, a fun place with a typical Montreal ambiance. It has a terrace outside in the back with real trees; inside, many floors with dance floors, pool tables, bars.

We drank beer and sangria, and my brother's friends all
thought I looked gorgeous! My brother was so happy to see
me smile again! Even though I did not believe my brother's
friends, their compliments made me feel like a woman again.
My feminine aura was back! I laughed so much that night.
One of my brother's friends even flirted with me. I could not
believe this. I thought he was making fun of me. I found out
later he was really flirting! Gosh. A breast missing, no hair on
my head, and this guy is flirting with me. Not that the guy
mattered to me – it was just the fact itself that mattered. Can
you imagine? Believe me, I slept like a baby that night. For
the first time in a very long time, I felt alive again. I was a
woman again. Wow!

The opportunity presented to Chantal by her brother was like
the giant's sword. It lay within reach, but it was up to Chantal to
grasp it and use it to slay her despair. She described the experience
as a turning point.

     I started to see some light in the closed sky and it gave
me the hope blue skies would return. I had to start a whole
process of loving myself again. A long, long, long road, and
certainly not the easiest one, either!

When Chantal was in hospital recovering from her surgery, one
of the nurses had said to her: "You can't wear anything sexy any
more. The bras will be bigger and so you won't be able to wear anything low-cut." The "rocker" jacket experience enabled Chantal to
reclaim her womanhood. Afterwards, she went out and found
camisoles that were lower and sweaters that were tighter than the
ones she used to wear. Through those acts of defiance, she
redeemed her former flair and won her femininity back from cancer. Her cancer recurred in 1999, and she went on Tamoxifen,

which caused her some weight gain. But changes in her body did not affect her sense of femininity. Once she won it back, she redeemed it forever.

🖊 Some of those sexy things I cannot wear, because I would look funny in them since I did gain some weight, but I don't give up. I'd rather be a bit chubby and healthy than skinny and sick!

Evelyn came to the brink when she found that she couldn't get into the program at Sudbury. The Sudbury doctors had given her a couple of names of doctors in the U.S. who could perform stem cell transplant operations, but this sword was not within reach. The operation would cost a lot of money, and neither Evelyn nor her husband could afford it. Her options were exhausted. The dragon sat on her chest. And then, out of the blue, Evelyn got a lucky break.

🖊 A lady who was a friend of a friend, who just happened to have had a bone marrow transplant several years prior, called me and asked me to please give her oncologist a phone call. She hoped that he might be able to help me. Well, I was reluctant to do this because Sudbury had told me that I wouldn't qualify anywhere else in Canada for a transplant, but I called just the same.

My new friend's doctor gave us the names of two doctors who worked at a hospital in Ottawa. When I called these two doctors, they agreed that I should go to Denver, Colorado, and that I should find out all that I could about the procedure – even bring them back the protocol – and upon my return they would see me in Ottawa.

So, I did exactly what they suggested, and after much persuasion they agreed to go ahead with the procedure in Ottawa – a procedure they had never done before. They did stem cell transplants for non-Hodgkins lymphoma, but they had never done a stem cell transplant for breast cancer – let alone a stem cell transplant with purging.

After almost a year of standard chemotherapy, I had a stem cell transplant with purging in December 1995. I am still in remission today – a miracle in itself.

Like Chantal, Julie and Evelyn, many of the women recalled that when they reached rock bottom, something extraordinary happened. Salvation came from an unlikely place; an unexpected opportunity was presented to them, but it required a deep act of strength. Evelyn's opportunity seemed to come out of the blue, a tip from a person she hardly knew. Chantal's opportunity came from her brother and his friends. These were serendipitous events; minor but momentous acts of grace. They required only that the women "reach for the sword."

Their lives could have gone one way or another. Evelyn might have ignored the opportunity, or it might not have arisen in the first place. Her fate lay in the balance, and for some reason, she had been spared. As Beowulf said when he returned to court after surviving the deep waters, "The risk was enormous, our encounter would have ended at once if God had not guarded me."

New Awareness

Beowulf emerges from the water a changed man. When he returns to court, the old King Hrothgar expresses what the hero already understands. He reminds Beowulf that he was not entirely responsible for his victory. He was saved by grace – and ironically, it was the dragon's own sword that saved him. Next time he may not be so fortunate. At court, King Hrothgar advises Beowulf to remember his mortality and

never become the victim of pride. Through battles with illness or
simply with age, even heroes with supernatural strength die, he says.
Soon enough "the gleam of eyes shall pass away and be darkened;
on a sudden it shall come to pass that death shall vanquish thee,
noble warrior."

The survivors emerged from the dark waters changed, deeply aware that the battle could have gone either way. While they had shown superhuman strength, spirit and determination, they were also profoundly humbled by the realization that their fate had not been entirely in their own hands.

No matter how well the battle has been fought, breast cancer can – and often does – return. It can recur or, worse, metastasize. A recurrence is a local event that happens either in the original site or nearby, in a different area of the breast. If the cancer metastasizes, it means that it has shown up elsewhere in the body – in lungs, liver or bones – and the chance of a cure is slim.

It was not easy for the survivors to live with the possibility that their cancer might return at any time. Yet there was no escaping the reality: their co-existence with the dragon was a fact of life. Marjorie Greenwood was diagnosed when she was in her late 60s, and she had a very rough ride. She and her husband had recently moved to Toronto, and she knew very few people there. She had her surgery in 1992 during a time when there was a shortage of nurses, and her care seemed haphazard. But Marjorie fought her way to recovery in spite of her aloneness and in spite of the system. She got through radiation, put herself on a macrobiotic diet, and was all set to put the nightmare behind her. She believed she had finally won her battle with cancer, once and for all. Then one day she called a woman who had been recommended by her surgeon as a "helper." Marjorie was eager to tell her helper the good news that she had recovered at last.

❧ I called her to tell her it was all over and I was fine, but she said, "Oh no, my dear, it is not over, ever." And so on. Amazingly, I did not know the cancer could recur, or metastasize! What a ninny I was then. I felt despair such as I had never known.

Marjorie had a tough time coming to terms with the fact that the dragon of cancer would be breathing down her neck for the rest of her life. Her profoundly discomforting realization was one that all the survivors struggled with. Marian found it very difficult to live in the "shadow of the dragon," haunted by the continual reminder that the dragon could spring out from nowhere at any time. But one day things changed.

❧ I was walking in the fall sunshine in a park near my home. The fall leaves had just started to turn. I was tired, stressed out and overwhelmed, wondering how I would ever make it through this predicament – if I would make it. In a blinding flash of insight, I realized that everyone dies. At some point, we will all die. The fact that I had cancer did not mean that I was immune from all other forms of death.

This may seem harsh and a bit trite, but it was an important realization for me. We all live in the shadow of death.

Cancer is a chronic illness, a disease that conditions life forever. For all their involvement in their survival, the women came to understand, as Beowulf did, that death was inevitable. This humbling realization forever changed the women's attitudes to life. Life became a wondrous, unpredictable journey, and every moment transformed into gold.

Beowulf emerged from the watery depths a changed man. He understood that the most noble warrior is not entirely in charge of his destiny. Fate had been kind – this time – but he was compelled to wonder, *Why was I saved?* It is an old question. But as King Hrothgar noted, the important lesson is humility. It is pride that puts us to sleep and severs our contact with what is real. "How deeply the soul's guardian sleeps," he said, when we are "enmeshed in matters of this world." An encounter with death awakens the soul and puts it back on watch, full of wonder and humility.

Having survived the underworld, the woman returned to the land of the living with new eyes. In his book *Myths, Dreams and Mysteries*, Mircea Eliade describes the initiate as one who can "see in the dark, literally as well as figuratively, for now he is able, even with eyes closed, to see through darkness and see things and events of the future, hidden from other points of view." The Inuit call the initiated shaman *elik*: "He who has eyes."

Keen eyesight is a universal characteristic of the dragon. The dragon's very name means "sharp-sighted." The word has its origin in the Greek word *drakon*, connected with *derkomai*, which means "to see" or to be "sharp-sighted." In fairy tales and legends from east and west, the dragon is the one who sees what the human doesn't see, or avoids. But when initiates go below ground to wrestle with the monsters of the deep, they emerge with the dragon's eyes. Not only can they see in the dark, but on every level they are awake, alert to the curious nature of destiny and the fragility of life. Whether the dragon is evil or good, writes John C. Lawson, whether it has wings or legs, teeth or talons, the universal characteristic of the dragon is that "it sleeps with its eyes open, and sees with them shut."

VI

The Heart of the Dragon

After he has conquered Grendel's mother, Beowulf returns to his homeland and becomes King. For 50 years he rules wisely over the peaceful land of the Geats. Then one day a man strays into the treasure barrow of a sleeping dragon, and he steals a golden cup. When the dragon wakes to find that he has been robbed, he is enraged. This dragon is a poisonous, winged fire breather, much feared by the land dwellers. He flies after the thief, scorching everything in his path. Unable to find the culprit, the dragon goes on a rampage and razes the King's abode, the seat of his hard-won throne. His life's work melts in surges of flame. This time Beowulf doesn't react as a warrior; he is overcome by grief. The senseless crime bewilders him. He wonders what he has done to deserve having his legacy destroyed in the late hours of a life lived so well and honorably. Old wounds and painful memories rise to the fore. Filled with sadness and loss, he travels to the dragon's barrow.

THE BIG SHOWDOWN

The worst scenario for any cancer survivor is metastasis, and no one can predict if and when this utterly lethal dragon will appear. Today, the average survival of women with metastatic breast cancer, from the time it first appears, is between two and three and a half years. Some women beat the odds and live for decades afterwards, but, as Dr. Susan Love writes, these are "rare and wonderful occurrences" and medical science has no idea what causes the cure in any of them.

The metastasis nightmare came true in Julie Davey-Prior's life. Julie's cancer first appeared in March 1995, when she was 38 years old. As a teacher in the Child and Youth Worker Program at Humber College in Toronto, she had been busy marking papers and looking forward to the end of the term. When she found the lump in her breast, a friend urged her to get an appointment and have it looked into. Her doctor thought it was just a fibroadenoma but made an appointment for Julie to get a mammogram. The image revealed a large lump close to the nipple, and the surgeon wanted to remove it so it wouldn't adhere to the nipple. No one was concerned about cancer.

Julie underwent surgery and awoke to learn that the lump was malignant and that her breast would need to be removed the following week. Her initial reaction was buffered by a Demerol haze.

> The next day the horror set in and I felt like I was living in the Twilight Zone. I kept waiting for the show to be over, but it persisted. I kept waiting to wake up from this nightmare, but it went on for days and days. Everything felt surreal. I could not feel the earth under my feet. Perhaps it was because of the river of tears that flowed from my eyes.

Julie described her dragon as a "fog dragon," a ruthless and powerful destroyer that came out of nowhere with a gaze focused singularly on her death.

> My dragon came out of the fog. He was sinister and sneaky, lashing out his venom when I least expected it. He was

untrusting and ruthless and filled with such immense power that he laughed at the thought of ever exposing himself and showing his gentler side. His victory was my death!

Before long, Julie and her partner, Rod, resolved to do battle with this formidable beast.

🌿 Within the first few days I remember Rod coming to me when I was sitting on the couch by the sun-filled window. He hugged me then looked me in the eye and told me that I was going to fight this thing. That I was not going to let it win. We were going to do everything in our power to overcome it. He was saying out loud what had just come to me that day.

The dragon roared!

I ended up having a mastectomy two weeks later. It was a sad parting. I loved my breast, and both of us honored it by saying goodbye and knowing that its sacrifice was to save my life.

Like the other survivors, Julie lost the feeling of invincibility; she mourned her lost breast and her lost choice to have children. She faced the dragon with courage, changed her eating habits, brought more balance into her life and reduced her workload for the first year while on chemotherapy. Meanwhile, she paused more often to smell the roses, and her relationship with Rod intensified.

🌿 We no longer took each other for granted. We held on to each other like never before. When life throws you into a tornado – that's what you do!

As Julie said, she could write for days about what she went through coming to terms with the cancer diagnosis: the fight, the tears, the chemotherapy, the healing, the support, and the challenges of living with a deadly disease. But she made her peace with her losses and carried on with her life.

In the fall of 1997, while she was still getting treatments, Julie saw a flyer for dragon boating posted on the wall at Wellspring, an emotional support center for cancer patients and their families. Julie loved to paddle a canoe on the lake at her cottage, and became excited about the prospect of paddling a dragon boat while she was in the city. In November, she met her dragon boat team. Pool practice began in the early spring and involved learning how to paddle by sitting on the edge of a swimming pool. Julie made the switch from a canoe to a dragon boat paddle stroke and enjoyed the experience of getting to know the other women. Then, in late April, the team went down to Toronto's Sunnyside harbor and she got into a dragon boat for the first time.

> We were all excited as we met at Sunnyside and entered the dragon for the first time. We were giggly and felt like children about to go for a thrilling ride. I was at the front of the boat, ready to pace for the right side. Beside me was a woman named Maria. How gloriously stimulating it was to make that boat glide over the water. It was a cool but beautiful evening and all our senses came alive to the splashing water, the grunts, the groans, the laughter, the cheering, the setting sun. And then the wonderful moment came when we got out of the boat and formed a line as we congratulated each other. This time-honored tradition of Dragons Abreast continues to be a highlight of our practices.

Julie loved dragon boating, and with her renewed strength she became a strong and powerful paddler for the first year and a half.

> I was a pacer and kept my focus on the front of the boat. I felt the power behind me but never saw it. At this point it wasn't clear to me that I was riding the dragon. For most of this time my dragon was back in the fog.

But in February 1999, two years after her diagnosis, Julie found a lump in her neck. The dragon had struck again – with even more deadly impact. The cancer had metastasized. It was in her bones, her lungs, her liver. "The reality I had learned to live with was nothing compared to the next stage of living life with metastatic disease," said Julie. She and her doctors decided to try a "hormone repressant" to see if the growth could be arrested. When spring came, Julie went back to dragon boating, but the dragon continued to make its presence known in the form of chronic back pain.

> 🌷The pain in my back was getting progressively worse, yet I was trying not to let it get to me. It was intermittent, and somehow I was able to carry on and push through it. When it wasn't there, I seemed to forget about it and live as if all were well. It amazes me that when I feel well, I forget I have cancer. But pain has a way of stripping you naked and leaving you vulnerable and fearful. Stopping the pain is all that you can concentrate on. Once gone, the clothes come back on and the smile returns. The relief from pain is a gift that you do not take for granted. The feeling of gratefulness is intensified.

Finally, in the summer, Julie was forced to stop paddling because of the cancer in her bones and the constant pain in her back.

> 🌷I knew that I could not paddle as I had in the past. I would not be able to give the 200 percent that a race demanded. I was scheduled to go to Vancouver with the team and I was overcome with sadness at the thought of not paddling. As luck would have it, our team needed a drummer. I willingly volunteered and the supportive encouragement from the team dissipated the sadness of not paddling. The team gave me the courage to sit up there before them and demand their attention. My focus became that of helping the crew to stay together and, in doing so, optimize their power.

The drummer plays a special role on the boat. She is the heart of the dragon, the motivational force of the paddlers. She beats the rhythm of the paddlers' strokes and keeps them all in time, moving as one.

🍃 The first time that I put my foot into the bow of the boat and straddled the mighty drum was in Vancouver. It was the day before the official races and the out-of-town teams were given the opportunity to practice in the unfamiliar water. It was a gray, overcast day with a great deal of dampness in the air. I remember feeling a chill, but it had more to do with my nervousness in this new role. I hugged the drum with my legs tighter than was necessary to maintain my balance in the wavy water. I remember feeling tentative at first as I recalled the words of our coach and brought the team to focus. But once I realized that they were depending on me to warm them up and take them through the race plan, I met the challenge and let my insecurities slip into the water. I knew what to do.

I sat up there and faced the strong and determined women before me who were prepared to give me everything I asked for. I felt their faith and trust in me. I felt and heard their support for me in my new role.

The drum was beautiful. I remember rubbing my hands over the skin and feeling the tightness of the stretch. It felt bigger than it looked from a pacer's seat. The wood of the drumsticks seemed to ground me. Their cylinder shape fit comfortably in my hand.

As a pacer, Julie had been used to sitting at the front of the boat, focused ahead, plowing her way to the goal. Now, as a drummer, her direction was turned around and she faced the women on the boat. While she kept them all in time, inspiring them to dig deep, she witnessed their power and determination, their intense and often painful effort to give everything they had. Drumming put Julie in touch with the women who made up the body of the dragon, and they filled her spirit with compassion and love.

🌿I see their focus. I see the simultaneous breath they take when they inhale the power of the dragon in preparation for a race. I see the pain of the push to give more and more as they approach the finish line. I see the relief and smiles on their faces when they hear, "Let it run!" at the end of the race. I see the excitement of a race well run. I see the tears of a fight well fought!

All through that summer, while Julie drummed, she hoped that the hormone therapy would work and she would slay the dragon. By August her hopes were high.

🌿We had taken over our friends' cottage for the summer, and overall I was feeling quite well and hopeful that the cancer would stop. I had been experiencing some back pain, but it was intermittent and I was able to ride it out. In August, we had some friends come up for the weekend and I had just purchased a portable hot tub, which added a great deal of comfort to the cooling evenings.

Rod had worked that week and arrived early Friday. We had a laugh fest with our friends that night, and in the morning as Rod and I cuddled, I started to talk about how grateful I was that I didn't have to be on chemotherapy. Then he told me. My oncologist had called and the recent tests showed that the cancer was progressing and that we needed to start a more aggressive treatment.

We both cried, and during the day I told my dear friends. That evening I experienced more back pain. The next day I experienced even more. It ruthlessly persisted. My friend offered me some Tylenol 3s. One didn't work. Two eventually did. Within two hours I was in more pain. I took more pills and got into the hot tub, which seemed to help on many levels. This continued all night. I would finally get some sleep as the pain abated, but two hours later I would wake in pain. In the middle of the night my grief overwhelmed me. Tears turned into sobbing, sobbing turned into wailing. The cancer was taking over. It felt like it was the beginning of the end. I was going to die.

Julie fought her metastasis hard, until she came to the limits of her strength and spirit. She realized that no matter how strong her spirit was, or how deeply she wanted to live, the dragon's will was stronger than hers. It just wouldn't go away, for all her heroic efforts.

🖋 At that time I didn't really feel there were any choices. Pain has a way of taking over, and easing it is all you focus on. We left for the city to see the doctor early Monday morning. I started chemotherapy that Tuesday. I ended up being on morphine, which was really hard for me, as I associated it with the end. I had palliative care radiation on my lower spine and began the process of weaning myself off the morphine.

It seemed to Julie that her powerful and vicious fog dragon would be content only with her death.

🖋 When he was weakened by drugs and laughter and hope and determination, he would slink back into the fog and hide. There he would harden his heart and develop devious plans to attack once more. His own wounds would fester and rot in his sunless hideaway until he could stand it no more, and then he would lash out again, feeling even more powerful as he brought me to my knees once more.

He was not prepared for my fight, and before long he was forced back into his fog lair, which had become even more unbearable for him. His own wounds fed his anger, and as it heightened he had to hit hard and furiously. But what kept him so angry? How did his venom continue to be so poisonous? How could he be more powerful than the drugs and the spirit that he was attempting to take? What could possibly stop this dragon from his ruthless pursuit of my death?

He did lash out, again and again and again. He filled me with cancer in my neck, my eye, my bones, my liver and my lungs. It became apparent that he was winning. I was weakening. Fighting him was not working.

So I befriended my dragon. He was hanging around and refused to go back to his home in the fog, so we got used to each other. I accepted him for what he was and began to live my life with him rather than against him. I started to look him in the eye, and in return I saw him softening. His blackened scales began to turn green, and in places they became iridescent and shone in the sunlight. Recently, I have noticed that his tail moves in a gentler way, his ears relaxed, his nostrils less flared, his roar softer, and sometimes it sounds as if he is purring.

Last week I received news that the cancer in my lungs is gone and that the tumors in my liver are shrinking.

Like the turn she made on the dragon boat, from paddling to drumming, Julie made a roundabout with her dragon. She entered a new relationship with her cancer, which she referred to as "dancing with death."

🌿 The new challenge has been to keep it at arm's length. Somehow in all of this I find I am making friends with the dragon. I hold the hand of death but somehow keep it turning and pirouetting away from me.

As Julie's story illustrates, the most courageous warrior spirit may still not be enough to slay the dragon. When Julie came to the limit of her strength, she changed her relationship with her cancer. She opened her heart to the dragon, just as she had opened her heart to the women on the boat. Such an act required facing the fury of the dragon not with vengeance but with love.

THE WOUNDED DRAGON

King Beowulf goes to meet the dragon at the barrow, and the two grizzled enemies face one another. Both have cherished the treasure they have protected, and both have been senselessly robbed. They are lashing out from the same wound.

While Fran was recovering from surgery, she observed that "the wounds of the dragon are our wounds."

> 🌿 On old charts, mapmakers used to draw a dragon where nothing existed. Indeed, a dragon was occupying the empty space in my heart. I was yet to make its full acquaintance. The dragon had been hurt in many ways. Its wounds were not even near healed, never mind acknowledged. It needed to become my friend.

Many of the survivors found that when they looked at their dragons compassionately, they touched their own wounds. Those who described their dragons in detail sometimes noticed that the creature wasn't always hostile; it had other hidden feelings and motivations. Julie Davey-Prior recognized that her deadly fog dragon had unseen wounds that "festered and rotted in his sunless hideaway." The more she battled her dragon, the angrier it became, and the more she suffered. The battle only escalated until she decided to change her response.

When Brenda Welsh depicted her dragon, she began to see that it was acting out of a wound that she could understand.

> 🍂 At times it was aggressive and would strike, causing great pain. Then at other times it was guilt-ridden and it would passively just wait in the distance with watchful and hurtful eyes. It had the ability to feel emotion and knew that it caused so much grief to so many innocent people, but had an uncontrollable need to continue its quest.

The more Brenda described her dragon, the more it became clear that the dragon's ruthless thieving came from a desperate need to have the thing it lacked.

> 🍂 When the dragon left, I could see it retreating back to its home with a part of my flesh and my innocent dream cradled under its wing. It left me physically scarred and wounded. The dragon was not smiling or looking proud of its accomplishments, but rather saddened by its uncontrollable desire to take away something so precious to me.

As Brenda pursued her dream of having a baby, she came to realize that the dragon didn't necessarily want to destroy her dream; it just wasn't capable of controlling its own powerful instincts.

> 🍂 In the distance I could see the dragon slowly releasing its strong grasp and trying to revive my dream. Because the dream was so young and weak, it was unable to find the strength to recover. The dragon sat watching over it, hoping that the dream would revive so that it could somehow be returned to me.

When Brenda came to see that the dragon was not purely malevolent, she began to perceive the possibility that some new opportunity might come out of the loss, that the experience might be purposeful in some way.

Barb Chomski saw her fire-breathing dragon as a creature who grew out of the pain in her own heart, a pain that was deposited there through many hurts, made up of all the physical and emotional bruises she had suffered living with a violent husband. In her attempt to create a secure and orderly home for her children, she had buried her injuries.

> I think, trying to sustain some kind of normalcy, you push things down, you push your fears down, you push a lot of things down. You put on a false face, because you have to be someone else in your job and with your kids.
>
> Where did my dragon live? In my soul, in the center of my chest, in my heart. I can imagine that the dragon grew bigger and bigger with every hurt, like a strengthening heartbeat. It started small, but it grew over the last 15 years. It grew on all the things I kept inside. And eventually the dragon woke, and all those hurts erupted into poisonous flames.

Breast cancer brought to the surface many old wounds that had accumulated through the women's lives. Most of the survivors said that the disease was a catalyst that forced them to reckon with deeply buried hurts and injuries. Akky, who volunteered at Willow, an outreach center for breast cancer patients, said:

> With breast cancer, everything comes to the surface. I see this in the calls I get at Willow. People are dealing with bad marriages and all kinds of deep problems. One woman I talked to had had several heart attacks, but she hadn't yet *experienced* her unhappiness – maybe because we think a heart problem can be fixed. But for many women, breast cancer is a death sentence, so everything comes up.

Some of the survivors said that their cancer arrived at a time when they were ready to deal with traumas and losses that they had sublimated in order to survive. Their dragons arrived at a timely hour to wake them up. Karen's dragon watched her from "on high," in the clouds or the treetops, while she went through a series of stressful events. In her mid-40s, Karen had been dealing with an aging mother, the loss of a close friend, the divorce of her parents and two school-aged children.

> 🕮 A year prior to diagnosis, I lost one of my closest friends to skin cancer. I never knew how sick she was till it was too late. My mother was not well. We were in the process of moving her into a nursing home. She had been having a series of mini-strokes that left her in bouts of depression. My sister Jane and I were doing the banking, grocery shopping and meal preparation for her. She had left my father at the age of 75 and now, 10 years later, was very dependent on my sister and me. I loved her very much, but I also had two boys at home, one five and one eleven, and a full-time job teaching a combined grade one/two, and I had just transferred to a new school and been given a very challenging class. I was a fully fledged member of the sandwich generation.
>
> In March of 1995 my dragon came leaping out of nowhere – out of the clouds – terrifying, uncontrollable, biting and nipping and all-consuming. It was there to carry me off, away from those I loved. It was huge and in complete control. I have difficulty describing it because I think that I was so frightened, I was afraid to open my eyes.

But when she did open her eyes, Karen saw the world anew.

> 🕮 Perhaps I had not opened my eyes to the life I was leading but simply going from day to day just surviving. Hence my wakeup call. Opening my eyes and waking up was like waking

up from the dream I was living and yet not really living…
I was not really happy with what was happening in my life.
I realized I wanted more!

Although Karen's dragon manifested itself as a fierce and hostile creature, her description of her relationship with it indicated that on some level it was intimately connected to her. It was not only watching but feeling those things she had not allowed herself to feel.

Chantal too described her dragon as a catalyst. It had been sleeping in a cave, quiet and undisturbed as long as her world was happy, the flowers were blooming, the insects buzzing and the children playing. But when she became discontented with herself and her life, the dragon grew restless and struck when she reached the depths of her misery.

> My "Dragon of Warnings" was a messenger from above that told me that my negative thoughts and feelings were hurting my own self. He looked miserable, unhappy and mean all at once. The Dragon of Warnings was not very big, nor tall. He did not hurt me in a way that I felt right away; the pain took time to be felt. He waited patiently until things got bad, and when the storm had been in the area for a while, the Dragon of Warnings came out of the cave where he lived and hit me like lightning.

Cathy had to tame her dragon with the determination of a bron-cobuster, but when she reflected on where it lived, she also came into connection with the wounded side of herself.

> My cancer dragon was very sinister and sneaky. I don't have a clue what it looked like, because I didn't see it coming. It struck so fast and unexpectedly and I didn't get a good look at it even then. I do, however, have a good idea where it had been hiding. It made itself a home in the most negative aspects of

my being, the spot where I complained about work, worried
about material things, and where I was caught up in sweating
the small stuff. I hadn't been exposed to too much big stuff,
so I expended way too much energy on things which I now
would think very little about. I try to keep that space in my
life very small now, so that no other nasty dragons will fit.

It is important to note that the women who recognized the
wounds of their dragons were not saying that they had caused their
own cancer, or that the cancer was the result of unexpressed
injuries. What they were saying was that the disease was a catalyst
that brought deep issues to the surface and precipitated a long-
awaited and sometimes even welcome catharsis. Those who came
to see their dragons with "soft eyes" found that the creature was
acting out of wounds they recognized. Like Beowulf facing the
dragon at the mound, they discovered that the dragon and the dragon slayer were not of two hearts, but one.

OPENING THE WOUNDS

*When Beowulf enters into battle with the treasure-guarding fire
dragon, he gets bitten in the neck. The poison soon causes the wound
to swell and fester. He stumbles around the barrow, delirious with
pain. It is not only the physical wound that torments him, but the deep
wound of losing everything he has built throughout his life. And under
that wound are still deeper wounds that go all the way back to his
childhood – crimes that he is powerless to avenge.*

Through the period of her cancer, Fran experienced many losses.
She lost two of her brothers, one to AIDS and the other to hepatitis.

And she lost her breast. The losses caused her to reflect on how attached we are to even the smallest piece of ourselves.

    🍂 As the Red River flooded its banks, many lost their homes and possessions. I grieved the loss of my little breast. As I prepared for mastectomy and tram flap reconstruction, I realized how wondrously we are made. The loss of a little bit of flesh, even in exchange for life, is a thing to be mourned and grieved. I was very sad, even knowing that life would go on, and "me" was essentially still there. But "me" was battered, and still facing surgery, recovery and chemotherapy.

It took time for Fran to absorb the full impact of what cancer meant.

    🍂 On the first impact, I thought cancer is a disease that can be treated medically and cured. I hadn't realized that this disease was an attack on my persona, my sense of well-being, on those intimate parts of myself.

Fran, who is an RN by profession, began to look at those attacks on her persona, the losses of body parts, of life, identity, relationships, femininity and womanhood. They leave a vacancy, she noted, and that gaping wound festers with grief, anger, despair and fear. For the wound to heal it needs to be opened, the poison drained and the wound cleaned. One needs to look into the pain and meet the anger, the fear, the grief; acknowledge it as a part of oneself and "treat" it with love, kindness and compassion. Because the wounds often have very deep roots, going all the way back to childhood, Fran advised proceeding gently, and at the same time fearlessly, moving towards the pain instead of struggling against it.

    🍂 I would like to make a gentle reference to the wounds that we all carry around from childhood, parts of oneself that need healing, angry parts of myself, unkind parts of myself.

I can treat those wounds by acknowledging those parts –
say, my unkindness. If I can say, this is a wound, it's not a beautiful part, but if I am able to uncover that wound, tear the
bandage off, I can treat the unkindness with a mental attitude
of compassion.

If situations that inflame the wound are met with kindness
instead of hurt or hostility, the wound begins to heal. And as we
treat the wounds, said Fran, they become "glorious." They "glow."
Pain becomes the very means through which to enter a place of
deep strength and compassion.

> ❦I have more compassion for those people who are unkind
> to me because I am in touch with my own unkindness. It goes
> with every part of oneself that is injured; the wounds caused
> by cancer become glorious. In befriending the dragon, you
> transform it.

Fran's cancer was a dragon that attacked like a "small but vicious
Rottweiler." Over time, as she uncovered and cleaned the wounds
that surfaced, it transformed into the dragon Fran now calls the
"Dragon of Glorious Wounds." It is a dragon inspired by Edward
Hays's book *St. George and the Dragon* – a companion who has
helped her to become more big-hearted and real.

> ❦He's a fun dragon, he's big, he's huge, he glows, he's beauti-
> ful. He's got a sense of humor, he's very human, he takes us
> right to where we are – with our husband, our kids, our
> anger, our hopes.

In Edward Hays's book, the Dragon of Glorious Wounds is a
tired old fellow with scarlet scales and great five-clawed feet
who invites the hero George on a quest. When George climbs onto
the back of the dragon, he notices that the creature's body is

covered with old scars and he limps now and again. George asks the dragon what the scars are and why they seem to glow golden-red in the dark. The dragon explains that they are old wounds, the wounds that accumulate through life. When the wounds rupture, says the dragon, "all hell breaks loose." The wounds holds us captive by telling us again and again how we were hurt and betrayed.

Then the dragon gives George the secret of transforming the wounds. He advises him to do the opposite of what the wounds tell him to do. If they say, "Run away," stand your ground. If they say, "Distance yourself," get close. Then, says the dragon, you transform them into a source of great power, great heart.

When Fran joined the Winnipeg dragon boating team Chemo Savvy at the age of 62, she found herself in the midst of many other women who, like her, were scarred. The day of her first workout, she walked into the gym to find 50 other women who were "glowing."

> Each woman was so vibrant. Each woman smiled. Each, whether age 35 or 65, was working out with might and main.
>
> Some scars were obvious – a cap or bandanna on a smooth head, a depression where a breast once rounded, a compression sleeve on a vulnerable arm. Other physical scars were well camouflaged. Emotional scars were temporarily forgotten or already being transformed into quiet strength. Words of encouragement were quickly offered. An occasional story was told in capsule form. "Wait until you get on the water!" the women said. The bonding was palpable.

When Fran took to the water with her dragon boat sisters, she began to ride her "Dragon of Glorious Wounds," gaining the physical strength and the power of compassion that came from digging deep for strength and meeting pain with love. Her description of a race reveals how she experienced the power of the dragon.

That lovely June evening that Crew Two first took to the boat, the water of the Red River was so brown and warm. My scarred body reveled in the thrust of paddle. I felt like the cliff swallows, aerodynamic and missioned, free to zoom from the dark nest of recovery to the bright flights of new life.

"Paddles Up! Take it away." Now I can skirmish with a physical adversary instead of the cancer bogeyman. "One, two, three, four, five, six." Now in the company with beautiful, strong women, I can dig into *this* battle. "UP, UP, UP, four, five, six, seven, eight, nine, ten, READY and REACH." Who would have thought that 22 wounded women could make 2,000 pounds of boat fly up so readily?

"Stroke! Stroke! Stroke!" We've got rhythm! We've got sync! Your strength is my strength. My strength is your strength. Together we can cope!

"SERIES IN THREE, TWO! ONE!" I can dig deep. I've dug deep before and struck the flowing springs of the healing spirit. ONE, TWO, THREE, FOUR, FIVE, SIX, SEVEN, EIGHT, NINE, TEN, READY AND REACH. My arms are getting tired. I'm breathing hard. But I am here. My body is responding like that of a young girl. I am with fabulous ladies. Can't let them down. Stroke! Stroke! Hope! Hope!

"Power in three! Two! One! POWER, POWER, POWER!" Where did this power come from? It is a gift. It is the power of one. It is the power of all. It is the strength of the group! It is the strength of the spirit! It is the strength of the one, weak from chemicals, but still here cheering on the riverbank. We are riding the Dragon of Glorious Wounds.

"We're almost there." My arms are weak. Shorter strokes. Deeper strokes! Harder strokes! Power strokes! There is always something more, even when I think I have given all. Scars are keloid tissue – tough – like a dragon. Injury, assault, produce strength. My spirit has been battered, but has healed stronger, gentler, warmer. The wounds are beginning to glow.

"Let it ride." The end of a practice, the end of a race. "Good job, ladies." Yes, let it ride! Who knows what one has really accomplished? Who will *really* know until all the results are in? That's the way it is with cancer – the way it is with dragons. But we have done battle, done it well.

We have allowed ourselves to know our injuries, know our pain, know our weaknesses, know our losses. In knowing, we have tended the wound. We have battled fear. We have battled loss. We have tended our weakened bodies and spirits. We have learned to embrace our pain. We are becoming "wounded healers."

Instead of trying to be like St. George and actually slay the dragon of illness and evil, we have responded to the invitation of the Glorious Dragon, acknowledging our wounds and weaknesses, and in graceful battle we have allowed them to glow. Our very wounds become the healers of our own spirit, for each other, and all those who cheer us on.

Now that I am a "dragon boat sister," I am no longer as concerned about my own cancer journey as I am for each woman with me. My heart breaks for the young woman who has lost her fertility, or who is afraid to become pregnant after treatment. I am so disappointed for the friend who has found a lump in the other breast or who has been told of a recurrence. I walk with those who journey with metastases, and pray that they be spared the "terrors of the night." My "glorious wounds" allow intimacy and empathy.

At a certain point in the battle with cancer, the warrior tires, or surrenders, or wonders, or becomes bewildered and confused. Like Beowulf stumbling around the barrow, the warrior cannot find anyone to blame, or anything to attack: there is only the injury. This is the point at which the survivors turned inward and made contact with their own wounds. Many recognized this as an opportunity to feel their own feelings, experience their own pain. As they healed the wounds, they began to glimpse the new possibilities – the treasure – that lay buried within the experience.

Gifts of the Dragon

In the final hours of his life, Beowulf asks his companions to take him down into the barrow so he can see the ancient store of treasure lying below. "Haste now," he says, "that I may see the old riches, the golden treasure, may eagerly gaze on the bright gems of artful work, so that, after winning the great store of jewels, I may more easily leave life and land, which long have I guarded."

Like Beowulf, who went down into the barrow to gaze upon the treasure that was now his, the women began to glimpse and to claim the gifts, the new opportunities and directions that emerged out of their ordeals with cancer.

Brenda Welsh and her husband did realize the dream of having a baby. It didn't happen the way they had originally planned, but their wish was fulfilled. In the summer of 2000, they got approval to adopt a little girl from China. As Brenda said:

> ❦ It took a long time for the dragon to return with our dream. It did not enter through the door but through a window. It will never be the same in our home since the dragon arrived, but we are all on the mend and have survived the fight. Now we are prepared to continue in a different direction.

Brenda would never have planned to go to China for a child, but as she came to accept the new direction offered by the dragon, she began to appreciate the possibilities and gifts inherent in the experience. It was perhaps a better destiny than the one she had planned, with many unforeseen rewards.

> In some ways I feel fortunate. I know that may sound silly, but so many positive things have happened to me since my diagnosis. I have gained a deeper understanding of myself. Several of my friendships have strengthened and I have developed some wonderful new friendships. I have become an advocate for the Breast Cancer Foundation and had the opportunity to be the guest speaker at the Run for the Cure in the fall of 1999. That was an amazing experience.
>
> I will be going to China soon to adopt a little girl. I look so forward to giving her an opportunity to achieve her goals. The chance to help out a little girl who is disadvantaged in some ways parallels my life. Because she was born female, she was more at risk of being orphaned, just as I was more at risk of getting breast cancer. I feel that I will be a better parent because I have gone through this challenge and hopefully will be more prepared to help my daughter deal with the difficulties in her life. I also feel that by challenging the Ministry of Community and Social Services' position on adoptive mothers with breast cancer, I am helping to pave the way for other women who are in a similar situation.

For Barb Chomski, the gift that came out of her illness was the opportunity to rest, recuperate and develop spiritually. For the first time in her life, she was able to take long, meditative walks, read spiritual books and gather what she had learned through the many ordeals of her life. She had such a craving for reflection and silence that Barb was inclined not only to accept but to embrace her cancer.

🌿 Where I was living, in Brampton, Ontario, at the end of the street there was a walkway, and I would walk through a patch of woods and come to a little stream with a bridge over it. When I paused at that bridge, I would always reflect on nature, and I would say a prayer.

First of all I would say, "Thank you." I was learning about appreciating, and I know it sounds weird, but I would thank God for giving me the cancer. Because it gave me the chance to look at my life, slow down. I really believe it was like a knock on the head. I was probably given the knocks before in the past, but I didn't see them. Now He said, "You're not listening. I'm going to hit you with a big one this time." So I would always pause on that bridge and I would say my thanks, and the sun would always come out. It never failed, even for a minute or a second. It never failed.

There were two red cardinals who came and lit on a tree. They were always there. I thought, *As long as I see those red cardinals every day, everything is going to be okay.*

More than a few women hesitated when they spoke about the gifts of the dragon. The idea that there might be anything redeeming about cancer is horrifying on first consideration. As Marjorie said:

🌿 I think having cancer is really, in a way, a gift. I know it sounds ridiculous, and when I first heard somebody say it I just about had a fit! My reaction was, "How can you say that? It's a terrible thing!" And I still think it's a terrible thing – I've lost friends to it. But it also opens vistas you never would have been open to, it opens your heart to others, and I've had some wonderful things happen to me since. Cancer has made me stronger. It made me less afraid to say what I mean and to stick up for myself – not take any guff.

On the other side of the spectrum, some women were adamantly not willing to give cancer the credit for the new opportunities that came out of it. Cathy was grateful for new friendships and experiences, and for deepened compassion, but from her point of view cancer was still a dragon that had senselessly robbed her and her friends of life.

> 🌿When I look back at what cancer has taken away from me versus what I have gained, it makes me angry. I have gained many wonderful things since my diagnosis, but I resent that the cancer should get any credit for it. What I have gained, though, are some very amazing new friends, women with whom I have journeyed through this cancer experience. It's hard to believe that I have only known the women from my support group since cancer, because the connection that we have is so deep. It feels as though we have been friends forever. Not only have I made new, amazing friends, but also I've come to realize how amazing are the ones I already have. I've also gained some new, important roles in my life. I spend time volunteering to help other women who are newly diagnosed with breast cancer, so that they don't have to make this journey alone. My professional life has also been improved. I work in health care and can say that I have a renewed commitment to my work, now that I've seen things from the other side. Truly the most important gain for me has been my involvement with the Chemo Savvy dragon boat team, and the wonderful women of this group.

It is hard to thank the illness for the unforeseen gifts that result from it, and yet we humans have a strange way of appreciating more fully what we have lost than what we have. Out of the emptiness of a loss we perceive the value of what we once took for granted. The old adage that "You don't know what you have until you lose it" applies here. Barb Chomski and some of the other women commented that they can get quite emotional when people say, "Ugh!" about having another birthday. For survivors of breast cancer, there is nothing sweeter than a birthday. Said Barb:

> ◊ When you live with cancer, you always have the fear that it is going to come back. The funny thing is that I can't envision myself being old. Now I appreciate every birthday so much more. When people get bummed out about their birthdays, I say, "Think about the alternative – *no* birthday!"

Interestingly enough, the French word "blesser" means "to wound." In Genesis 32:36, Jacob says to the angel who wounded him, "I will not let you go unless you bless me." It gives us pause to wonder if there isn't a blessing in every wound, if we are able to receive it. As Stephen Larsen points out in *The Mythic Imagination*, to receive the blessing we have to face sickness and suffering, and move into it, not away.

Burial

> *In the final moments of* Beowulf, *the conflict between the King and the dragon comes to an end as both succumb to their wounds. Before he dies, Beowulf asks that a tower be built in his name at the site of the barrow overlooking the sea. His last wish is to serve as a beacon to all ships passing in the night.*

At some point in time in the process of living with breast cancer, the survivors came to peace with the losses of cancer. They were able to bury their old dreams and identities. Brenda Welsh told the story of how she ceremonially buried the dream to have her own child.

In April 1998, after my chemotherapy and radiation were completed, I attended a retreat for breast cancer survivors near Sudbury. A wonderful woman named Cian, who was also a survivor, organized the weekend. It was hosted at a missionary retreat and was an extremely uplifting soul-searching experience. I participated in a healing circle, a native tea ceremony and a burial. We were given clay and told to mold it into something that we needed to let go. Mine was a tiny person which represented the child I would never feel growing within me.

After we all finished molding the clay, we marched up the hillside to a dug grave. It was a very cold day, somewhat fitting to the experience.

When we got to the grave site, we had the choice to say a few words or simply place the object into the ground. Women began sharing their stories as they placed their clay molds into the grave. Some women molded breasts and told of their need to put the cancer behind them; one woman talked of being sexually abused as a child and feeling relieved because she no longer had to keep the secret. Another woman talked of an unfulfilled marriage and her need to move on.

It was a very moving experience and we all cried a lot as we helped each other try and find peace within ourselves. When we were coming down the hillside I remember laughing with my friend Nancy and feeling that the weight was starting to lift from my shoulders.

While Brenda buried her old dream, Bernice buried her former identity – the identity that she had acquired to survive her difficult childhood. Bernice, who is Métis, grew up in Manitoba and was extremely protective of her younger brothers and sisters. Because of their nationality, the children had a tough time in school, and to make it worse, they came home to an atmosphere filled with tension and potential violence. Bernice developed a protective and withdrawn identity that she finally put to rest through her journey with cancer.

> ❦ The one I was burying was a shy and introverted lady who puts her head down when she's at home. I was burying the person who was ready to please everybody before pleasing myself. I was a people pleaser; I wouldn't make waves. I would go along with the group.

When Bernice buried her old persona, she embraced and redeemed the person whose needs had been sublimated in order to protect and care for her siblings.

> ❦ I'm living my life very differently since my diagnosis. I was always doing things for others – never saying no. I have tried my best to be there for anyone who needed me, whether I wanted to or not.
>
> Now I realize that *I need me!* I must look after myself first. Then if I want to do things for others (and I often do), I can, but if I have to alter my plans to accommodate them, I just say so. They are understanding, but I'm sure they're a little hurt at times too. But the new me comes first. The guilt isn't there when I say no and, best of all, I decide whether or not I wish to do something or go somewhere without asking for my husband's permission first! This is the biggest and best change I have made for myself. I'm not as fastidious in my housework these days. It gets done, but in my good time. I relax more and I'm enjoying life now more than I ever did, believe me!

Bernice felt that her benevolent dragon, who made its first appearance in her strong urge to get a breast screening, had been waiting all her life to emerge and carry her towards her true self.

🌿 I could not ever think of a dragon taking anything away from me – on the contrary. This dragon of mine entered my life just when he felt I could handle the shock and grief of being diagnosed with this cancer. He gave me another chance at life, and had he not awakened when he did, who knows?

He gave me courage to stand up for myself and make choices that I felt were right for me – and above all, to be my own person.

Through the grieving process the women slowly put their old lives, identities and dreams to rest. Some went to see grief counselors to help them through the mourning process. Akky sought the help of a therapist in order to put her role as a mother and nurturer to rest. In the process of laying down her former life, she came to see that though she had loved the role, she wouldn't want to repeat it. While on the outside she had a nice home, family and job, inside she had felt depleted, spent, invisible and unrecognized. When her children began leaving home, she had already started a process of dying. Before her cancer, it seemed to her that she had become an empty shell, "a stone ghost."

To Akky, cancer seemed like a confirmation that she had come to the end of her life. But in the course of coming to terms with her losses, she found that she was very, very afraid of death. One day, while in session with her counselor, the therapist asked her, "What is it about death that frightens you so much?" She thought about that. What really scared her was that she hadn't *lived*. She came to see that the one she had been missing all her life – herself – was the one she had the opportunity to live for now.

The Dragon Transformed

"There are two dragons in dragon boating," said Barb Chomski. On the one hand there is the dragon that is battled fiercely, the cancer, the adversary in Lane 11, the deadly water dragon that you beat down with all your might. On the other hand there is the dragon underneath you – the silent, unspeaking one who carries you forward, helping you to regain your strength and to heal. As Barb said:

> ⚘ One day I said to the girl beside me, "Imagine that there's cancer down in the water, and you take your paddle and you spear it." So you're slaying one dragon and, at the same time, the dragon is carrying you. He's the dragon boat, helping you to slay the dragon of cancer.

When Barb considered her personal dragon who lay in the fiord, breathing fire, she knew he was in the process of being transformed and one day she would find him beautiful. There would come a time when, through dragon boating and her own inner work, she would truly "ride the dragon."

> ⚘ He is a winged creature, red and gold, and eventually he will take off into that sky. I can imagine myself riding his back one day, when I've made peace with him.

Anita remembers the very moment she came to peace with her dragon. She had hardly got into the water for her first dragon boating practice when she began to experience a change in herself and her dragon.

> ⚘ Since both mastectomies, I'd never completely felt *good* about the disfigurement… had not really accepted it, I guess,

but always coped, 'cause that's what I do. The whole situation was mentally both bleak and black to a degree greater than I was truly aware.

Our first practice session took place in Victoria's Inner Harbour. Boy, were we novices! Trepidation quickly changed to empowerment with the sudden awareness that we were *doing* it! *This* was the turning point, undoubtedly.

Being an integral part of the paddling team, and powering the boat so silently yet so strongly, signified the beginning change within me. "If I can do this, what else can I do?" I was totally exhilarated after our first race the next day, and while physically exhausted, emotionally I could have taken on the whole Pacific Ocean! Talk about a high!

At this point the dragon became my savior. I fully realized, fully, how totally alive and strong I *still* was. I think a part of me had died previously and suddenly I felt whole again. The black dragon faded and rainbow colors replaced it in an instant. It's incredible how quickly the change took place. Acceptance washed over me.

Until that moment Anita had been struggling with "never-ending worry and anger over the unfairness of it all," but now her dragon changed from a destroyer to her own wise and beneficent personal ally.

〰 The dragon became this lady's best friend, an ally in my personal battle. He took something very bad away from me, something that had the potential to kill me; he was my savior. I guess he'd hung around until I really needed him. But, boy, he sure let me go through a lot first! So it goes with dragons, I suppose. I've never known one before.

Now I picture him as being turquoise blue, pink and green. Poor fellow, but those are my colors of trust and love. He has become *good*. He's helped me by giving me a second chance at living.

My old world had gone from some complacency (before diagnosis) to instability and uncertainty (after diagnosis). This new world has a better focus with a sense of acceptance, power and beauty, both within and outside myself. I don't hate my own disfigurement like I did before. Strange, but that's how I feel.

Franci remembered the moment when she came to peace with her dragon. In her very first dragon boating race, she was walking nervously down the pier towards the boat. She was still recovering from radiation, and the painful burn had begun to subside at last. As she approached the boat, she felt herself reaching out towards the head of her green-winged fire breather. In that instant she accepted the lifelong presence of her cancer. As she said, "I realized that the cancer could recur, but I was ready to ride that dragon."

🍃 I closed my eyes, took a very deep, long breath, held it for a moment and exhaled slowly, opening my eyes. I was still here – full of fear and consuming uneasiness. The ferociousness of the dragon had simmered completely. It appeared to be more of a misbehaved pup waiting to be scolded. I reached out cautiously and carefully. Then, touching its head, I accepted it. After that it was a matter of building trust and coming to terms with the fact that the dragon was going to be a part of my life, a part of me. This permitted me to lift my head high, stare down the dragon and get close enough to gently climb on for "the ride"!

During their healing process, those women who depicted deadly dragons found that as they changed, so did their dragons. Their dragons became benevolent, redemptive beings who possessed the wisdom of their true destinations. As Akky began to pursue her dreams, her dragon transformed from a malevolent, secretive enemy to a beautiful creature, sometimes solid, sometimes vaporous, who could carry her to dimensions both physical and imaginative. Wherever she got off track, the dragon was there, underneath her, to bring her back on course.

> ✹ My dragon is very friendly. It's mystical. At times it's like vapor – it just disappears – and at times it's very clear and solid. It can take any shape or form and it can go anywhere. It takes me into the risky areas and the restful areas. My dragon is there when I need it... and when do I need it? When I'm not listening to my little inner voice, when I'm sidetracked with other people's important things which are not necessarily mine. My dragon is always there when I need to listen to where I need to go.

For some women, the dragon had always been kind. They could not make a link between their cancer and a dragon. Their dragons were emergent: they signified the guidance and the opportunities that came out of the cancer experience. They introduced them to a different dimension of life, opened their eyes to its wondrous and mystical aspects. They embodied the women's delight, their gratitude and the almost childlike wonder that they experienced when they emerged from the ordeal. Their lives may have been cut short by the disease, but the benevolent dragon had carried them through, strengthening their spirits and opening their eyes and their hearts.

At first, Evelyn couldn't imagine what her benevolent dragon looked like, although she felt its presence on the water and in her life. As it turned out, mystery was the mark of her dragon, an elusive creature who gave her glimpses into the truly supportive and wondrous nature of life.

My dragon is neither fierce nor friendly – neither friend nor foe. Joseph is the name of my dragon, and he can best be described as a spiritual entity. He is a mysterious dragon and wears a coat of many colors. Just as a rainbow requires certain conditions to appear and exist, so does my dragon. When and if my dragon is to be seen, he appears as an object of both beauty and wisdom, staying only a short while before he vanishes, as if into thin air.

Joseph, my dragon, has touched my life in ways that I never thought possible. He has given me a multitude of brief moments that can only be described as beautiful. These moments, like a rainbow, appear only when the conditions are right.

I never thought much about dragons before my cancer diagnosis. Mostly, I thought dragons were dark, lurking creatures, certainly not things of beauty and wisdom. Now I look for dragons all the time, mostly in shopping malls, stores and dragon boat festivals.

At first I couldn't see my dragon, but not too long ago my close friends on the dragon boat team bought me a beanie baby dragon to take with me when I go to Ottawa for my radiation treatment, and it was then that I realized its significance. I thought to myself, "That's it – that's my dragon." It was my Joseph dragon with a coat of many colors, a striped belly and angel-like wings on top of his head.

I now have respect for the dragon which I never had before. I look for those brief moments when the dragon appears, and I cherish those beautiful moments in all their glory and splendor.

Kaethe Lawn was reticent at first about describing her benevolent dragon. Although she felt a connection to this strangely thrilling and vital symbol of dragon boating, it took a bit of a leap to start writing about it. But as soon as Kaethe began pulling her dragon out of the ether, it sprang to life. It began as the "mascot of the team" but soon took on a life that was hers alone.

> As our team mascot I could picture a well-mannered, friendly dragon, the size of a small crocodile. She would have a strong, toned body with multicolored scales, each one shiny and well formed. Her body would be carried by sturdy, stubby legs and five-toed feet. Her jaws would curve up at the edges (like a cat's) so that she would always have a pleasant smile on her face. Her eyes would be golden and display intelligence and affection. When she would like attention, she would mew with an alto voice and gently wave her tail from side to side while looking up with expecting, trusting eyes.
>
> It would be a joy to have her around and she would be in the boat with us during training and races, encouraging us through her presence. At night she would go home with the team captain and rest underneath her bed. There would be a soft blanket for her, of course, but even then the scales of her body would make a gently rattling noise when she changed position in her sleep. The team captain has told us that she likes to hear her easy, relaxed breathing and her occasional (*very* occasional) soft snoring.

Coming into the heart of the dragon is a story of acceptance. The women who struggled against the dragon of cancer ultimately went from trying to kill it to accepting it, and when they did, their hearts opened. As they greeted the dragon, they greeted themselves. Their stories suggest that the dragon is the ultimate stranger, the unwelcome guest who comes knocking on our door and refuses to be turned away. The women who entered the heart of the dragon received that guest. As we read in *A Course in Miracles*:

> ❦ Your Guest *has* come.... You did not hear Him enter, for you did not wholly welcome Him. And yet His gifts came with Him. He has laid them at your feet, and asks you now that you will look on them and take them for your own. He needs your help in giving them to all who walk apart, believing they are separate and alone. They will be healed when you accept your gifts, because your Guest will welcome everyone whose feet have touched the holy ground whereon you stand, and where His gifts for them are laid.

When the women entered the heart of the dragon, their struggle with the disease ended, which doesn't mean that the cancer went away. The threat would always be with them. What it means is that the struggle against themselves ended; the slayer and the enemy "died" together. The women came to see that even death was not against them. It was in a mysterious way bringing them closer to themselves, closer to home. So began a cooperation that transformed the deadly dragon into a beautiful companion and the dragon slayer into a brave and gentle rider, humbled by the mystery of life.

VII

Riding the Dragon

TAKING THE REINS

While Beowulf and the poet Qu Yuan met their fates differently, both their spirits survived death. As Qu Yuan relates in a poem, after he left his life behind, he seized the reins of the jade dragons and began a new journey.

> *Many a heavy sigh I heaved in my despair,*
> *Grieving that I was born in such an unlucky time,*
> *I plucked soft lotus petals to wipe my welling tears*
> *That fell down in rivers and wet my coat front.*
> *I knelt on my outspread skirts and poured my plaint out,*
> *And the righteousness within me was clearly manifest.*
> *I yoked a team of jade dragons to a phoenix-figured car*
> *And waited for the wind to come, to soar up on my journey.*

Many women described their lives after cancer as a spiritual journey, and they related deeply to Qu Yuan's redemption by the spirit dragons. The poet's story was their story too. As Irene Hogendoorn, a member of the Toronto team, said:

> Qu Yuan was a lost soul; he was spiritually drained. Cancer patients are like that. They have to deal with the "brutal warfare" that takes place within their bodies as they attempt to

rid themselves of the evil. Cancer can leave one depressed and wandering aimlessly, but when you contact the magical, powerful dragon, like the ones in Qu Yuan's poem, you wait for the "wind to come and to soar up on your journey."

I was drained, but I was saved!

Pamela said:

🌿 I relate to the poet's banishment and heavy-heartedness. The lesson for me is to wait for the wind to come and let the dragon take me where it will.

And Julie Dubuc said:

🌿 The rock represents the trauma of dealing with a diagnosis of cancer. It can drown you if you don't let go of it. Hitching my car to a pair of jade dragons represents my decision to join Chemo Savvy and take up the reins of my life.

For most of the women, dragon boating was the vehicle of their redemption. The benevolent dragon of the dragon boat appeared to them like the jade dragons of Qu Yuan, inviting them to begin a new way of life. They vividly remembered the magical means by which they had been drawn to dragon boating in the course of their recovery. Bernice had already made a connection with her dragon – her benevolent inner guide – before she encountered dragon boating. Then, a year after her diagnosis, Bernice had a dream in which her dragon appeared to her in the form of a boat, and let her know she was rounding the corner.

🌿 I was diagnosed early in 1997, and in the fall of that year I had a dream that I was in this very long boat. It seemed to me like there were a lot of people in the boat with me and we were all paddling. It was more like in a gondola – we all had these huge paddles. We were in a canal, and the buildings were floating by: tall buildings with lots of windows like those in Holland or Italy. The boat that we were in had a very ornate head, like a dragon's head.

Later in the fall, one of the members of Breast Cancer Action Manitoba brought in a video of the first race of Abreast in a Boat. I watched it thinking, *I've got to get into one of those boats!* not remembering the dream. Then we were asked, "Is anybody interested in forming a team?" And of course I was one of the first ones to say yes!

Driving home that night, I was humming to myself, thinking about the video I had watched and picturing myself in the boat, and all of a sudden it dawned on me that I had dreamed about this already! It was like a déjà vu. I got goosebumps all over, I was so excited. When I got home I was in awe! I could not get this dragon boating thing out of my mind. I had to paint a picture, which is what I do when something really important happens. I called it *The Turning Point*.

Dragon boating became a lifeline for the survivors. It helped them to recover physically, it provided their emotional support group and it was a symbol of their new identity, their new life. The challenge was to seize the reins of the opportunity and stay on for the ride. It was not always easy. The rigors of dragon boating required that the women make a commitment to themselves and their own recovery. For women who had defined themselves by their selfless service to others, dragon boating meant laying claim to a new identity. As Julie Dubuc said:

> I have always been one of those women who puts everyone else before themselves. I am the oldest of five children and pretty much raised my brothers and sisters. I have always believed that being of service is an honor and a privilege.
>
> But I came to see that helping others was a way of making

myself feel of value. That weighed me down and caused me to feel like I was drowning. I had to stop trying to make life as comfortable as possible for everyone else.

This is where my dragon boating team, Chemo Savvy, has really been of value. I am committed to going to my workouts, practices and races. It is one of the only things that I do where I absolutely put myself first... it has been good training for me. My family has encouraged me, rather than trying to dissuade me, and I am pleased and flattered that they will sacrifice for me.

Brenda Tierney expressed a similar realization when she reflected on the legend of the drowning poet.

✺ The legend told me that it is important to be aware of your own worth. Other people can destroy your life if you let them. It is important to understand what you can change and what you can't change, accept it, and then continue to live your life. If you do not have goals in your life and do not maintain your sense of self and direction, life can seem meaningless. Despair destroys. All times have lucky and unlucky times; it is how you deal with those experiences that determines how you live your life.

Phoenix Rising

Qu Yuan described his chariot as a "phoenix-driven car." The phoenix has special significance for women who are dragon boating, because the "phoenix boat" specifically refers to a women's dragon boat. Furthermore, the phoenix is a universal symbol of redemption and immortality. The Egyptians believed that the phoenix lived in Arabia, where it returned every 500 years. It built itself a nest of spice branches, set it alight and expired in the flames.

After three days a new phoenix would rise from the ashes, herald-
ing the beginning of a new age or the rule of a great emperor. It has
been said that the phoenix feeds on dew and harms no living thing.
For the Chinese, the phoenix or "Red Bird of the South" was purported to know the whereabouts of treasure.

Each of the breast cancer survivors experienced a phoenix-like
redemption following the death of her former self. Out of the ashes
she rose, a new being with new eyes, a new awareness of her life and
her purpose. It was time to realize the many dreams buried deep
within her soul, and to come fully into herself during the time
remaining to her.

Many new opportunities came out of the survivors' ordeal with
cancer. After her illness, the Amazonian Helen Sharpe divorced
and then went to law school, where she reinvented herself as
a lawyer.

> You can knock an Amazon down, but you cannot knock
> her out. So I applied to and was accepted into law school.
> September 1977 was the beginning of a whole new and
> exciting chapter of my life. When I was called to the Bar
> in April 1982, I was almost 50 years old, and had become a
> grandmother for the first time!

At 53, Anita retired from her job as a mammographer and took
up creative writing, which spurred and regenerated her lifelong
mission as an educator.

> I signed up for the course and am really a published free-
> lancer now! I can speak freely and openly about myself, with-
> out crying, about almost anything that's happened in my life
> (but I still weep over our pet dog whom we put down three
> years ago). I have become even more committed to doing
> presentations about breast health care. Women *must* do it.
> It's that simple. My message is: "Look at me. I did it, and

maybe that's why I'm still alive today. The lump was only 4 millimeters. But I found it. You can, too."

When Akky emerged from her illness, she wanted to realize a dream that had been buried within her since childhood. She had grown up in Holland, close to an air force base, where she had watched training flights with utter fascination. Sometimes a plane would crash and Akky would see the black smoke rising from behind her house. "You would think that would have turned me off," she said, "but it didn't." Flying epitomized the most exhilarating and risky thing she could do.

〰 To me, the pilots in war stories were heroes. Flying was a dangerous thing to do. At 16, I wanted to learn to fly. I had taken up horseback riding – I loved that. One day I went up in a helicopter, and after I told my parents I wanted to fly. They said, "No way are you ever going to fly." From their point of view, people who have their pilot's license are the first to be conscripted into the air force, and during wartime their life expectancy is not long. To this day I still haven't told my mother I fly.

Before her cancer, Akky's dream remained in the realm of fantasy. From time to time she would go out to Toronto's Pearson Airport, sit in the restaurant sipping a coffee and watch the planes go by. But when she was recovering from cancer, her wish to fly became urgent and real. She found herself going out to a smaller airport nearby.

〰 I went to the Buttonville airport just to have a look, sit out on their patio and think about flying, and one day I was sitting there and I thought, *What am I doing just thinking about it? I'll just sign myself up for the ground school, just to have a chance to learn about it.* So I signed myself up for the ground school.

It didn't make sense to go to ground school and never go up in the air, so when someone suggested that Akky take flying lessons, she seized the opportunity to do it.

> ‼ I took the risk of learning to fly. This seemed such a strange and foreign world to me, but I took the plunge and signed myself up. I could no longer put it off. The world of aviation opened up to me. Flying took me outside of my home to new places, where I met new people at all hours of the day and night. Some of the training was so indescribably exhilarating, and some maneuvers, like stalls and spins, were pure terror.

When the survivors took hold of their goals, they often met with resistance from those who were unsettled by the changes they were making. Akky's husband, Henry, didn't want her to fly because it was too expensive and, furthermore, too risky. But his concerns did not block Akky.

> ‼ When I started training, it involved learning risky maneuvers, like stalling the plane or doing a spin or spiral. You need to learn these things so you can get familiar with all the attitudes of the plane. When I came home and told Henry what I had done, he said, "I don't want you doing that any more."
> "Well, that's what you have to do to get your pilot's license," I said.
> "Well, I don't want you getting a pilot's license," he said.
> I went ahead and did it anyway.

As it turned out, when Akky went forward and Henry saw how determined she was, he got behind her and in fact became her greatest supporter and fan. She kept on going, meeting one obstacle after another. Getting her pilot's license also required passing a medical exam, and now it was the aviation doctor who stood in her way.

The aviation medical doctor wasn't that keen on me getting a license. He said, "Have you dealt with all the issues that go along with having a body part amputated?"

I thought, *What would be the issues? The loss, the mourning?* He was afraid the cancer would metastasize. I thought, *I don't need this guy in my life*, so I found another doctor.

Whatever they aspired to do in their new lives, whether it was dragon boating, flying, creative writing or law, the survivors had to be very firm about their dreams and ventures in order to stay on course. Like the steersperson in a dragon boat, they faced the challenge of keeping their eyes on the destination while meeting the conditions of wind and water with flexibility.

For some it was rough going at first, because they met with resistance just at the time when their dreams were still fragile and embryonic. Bernice's husband was not in favor of her dragon boating, but Bernice recognized that she needed to pursue her dream no matter how he felt about it. When she finished her painting *The Turning Point*, she asked the team members to sign it, and then she had it framed. She was proud of her painting. It had demanded considerable effort and courage for her to get every woman's signature on it. She hung it over the sofa in the living room, but her husband wanted her to take it down. Cancer and dragon boating continued to be sore points for him and he didn't want to be reminded of them every day. Bernice obliged, but meanwhile the painting became so popular with her team that cards were printed as fundraising items. Before long, team members were requesting prints so they could hang the picture in their own homes, and the original went up in a public place: Winnipeg's Breast Cancer Centre of Hope.

In her gentle way Bernice conceded to her husband's resistance, but at the same time she did not stop dragon boating or painting pictures inspired by the sport. While she was hurt that the painting could not hang in her own home, she understood that her husband's struggle for control had deep roots. She hoped that in time he would come round, that he too would heal, and she was not disappointed.

> ❧ Just recently, oh, about three weeks ago, he actually sat down and watched a whole program on breast cancer survivors with me. We usually sit and have coffee in the morning and the program came on. He said to me, "Do you want to watch this?" and I said, "Yeah." I assumed he would take his coffee cup and walk away, but instead he set it down and watched the whole thing with me! I thought, *My goodness, is the sky gonna fall?*

The way in which the survivors met resistance is interesting. While they kept faith with their dreams and goals, they responded to setbacks with the resilience of a pilot who is adept in the wind and the water. They gave in when it was necessary and found another way, but they never gave up. There were times, however, when they were almost overwhelmed. Akky, who had learned how to fly an airplane, later became a steersperson for the Toronto dragon boating team. Her training in the air had taught her to be calm in a crisis and to utilize the maneuvers she had learned. But when she started dragon boating, she discovered a whole new set of challenges, which were not only mental but physical and emotional. In fact, her first race experience was so emotionally charged that she nearly quit dragon boating.

> ❧ When I started steering the boat, I feared that I wouldn't be good enough or strong enough; I wouldn't be able to steer the boat straight or maneuver it to the start position of a race correctly. This has been a lifetime problem of mine, that of not feeling adequate or good enough – not valuing what I do and waiting to be criticized for it.

After the first race one of the members blamed me for losing the race. She shouted, "Let's get rid of Akky!" after she got off the boat.

I really doubted my skills and wondered if the team would be better off without me steering. I was hurt and disappointed. I didn't need criticism when I was trying to build my self-esteem. I felt alone out there and completely exposed. As a steersperson I stand at the back of the boat and stick out like a sore thumb. If I make a mistake, everyone knows and the whole team suffers. All my life I have lived in the background and worked on not being noticed and staying out of trouble. I feared being criticized and now I had put myself out in the forefront, exposing myself to the world.

She thought about quitting but recognized that "that was the old me." Her new phoenix spirit was calm in the face of opposition and didn't want her actions to be dictated by her emotional wounds. So she examined the remark her teammate had made. It was surely unkind, but was there anything useful in it?

〰 It was sort of a turning point because at first I thought, *Gee, for the sake of the team maybe I should step down. Maybe my voice isn't loud enough.* Then it dawned on me. It isn't just a loud voice you need to be a good steersperson; you've got to have a race strategy, steer the boat, do all the other things as well.... So I thought, *Louder voice, well, I can work on that.* So I recruited Marjorie Greenwood, who is an actress and former drama coach, and we went to a church and worked on projecting my voice.

So now if the team can't hear me, I know that it's not just me, that it's the wind and the water, other people shouting, other conditions. I never did before. I never turned a problem around and saw my responsibility and others' as well.

The survivors undertook to fulfill their dreams with the same fearless realism and persistence they had gained by meeting their cancer. The events that had once caused them to flinch and withdraw were the very shadows that they learned to face and move through. As they kept faith with their dreams, they began to ride the dragon; and dragons, it seems, have long been known as creatures who can fly through anything. They know the time to be still, to move forward, to shape-change or retreat, and so it is not easy to trap them. As Paul Newman recounts in his book *The Hill of the Dragon*, the philosopher Confucius once consulted his archivist, Lao-Tzu, and after the visit Confucius made the comment: "Birds fly, fish swim, animals run. The running animals can be caught in a trap, the swimmer in a net, and the flyer by an arrow. But there is the Dragon; I don't know how it rides the wind or how it reaches the heaven. Today I met Lao-Tzu and I can say that I have seen the Dragon."

Riding the Dragon

"Dragon boating," said Evelyn, "takes me to a whole new dimension."

> It's a very spiritual experience. I hear our drummer, Julie, yelling, "Give me an inch!" and with that all 20 women reach out and you can feel that boat surging ahead. She then yells, "Not faster – long…er, deep…er." It feels like the boat is flying and, in fact, I'm sure that it is. It's poetry in motion.
>
> These moments are precious. I'm not thinking about anything except my stroke and the sheer love of the sport. Once in a while I glance around and take in the beauty, and I hear

one of the ladies yelling, "Look at the horizon, ladies, isn't it beautiful?" With that I look around and see a mysterious dark gray sky with this unbelievable golden horizon. Even more spectacular is the beauty of the rain as it pelts the shadowy water. We are all getting drenched, but we don't seem to mind because it feels like we are schoolchildren playing in the puddles. And the water, well, it just giggles at us, as each raindrop hits its surface and bounces off. I feel like I'm at some far-off mystical place, and with that I hear our drummer yell, "Let it run, ladies." Back to reality.

When the women "grasped the reins of the jade dragons," they entered a new, more spontaneous and creative relationship with life. With their old dragons they had slain the will to make things go a certain way and they had come to a realization that life has its own way. They would live out their dreams with will and intention and, at the same time, ride with the currents, borne on the winds of destiny.

Before her cancer, Barb Mitchell of Vancouver lived in a very controlled and managed way, and the years leading up to her diagnosis were emotionally draining. She had been extremely unhappy in her marriage, but she kept "burying the emotional losses" because she had three teenage daughters to raise and could not fathom how a divorce would be possible financially. With all her might she tried to hold things together, but eventually, inevitably, her marriage did come apart.

🌿 My husband was trying to start his own business and in the process we lost our home, our cars and all the emotional stability in our marriage. At two different times I quit jobs I enjoyed to help with the business, but in the end we still lost everything.

Nine months after she separated from her husband, Barb discovered her breast cancer. She had been aware of the lump for some time, but she had put it on the back burner until she was ready to deal with it. For Barb, who had been used to managing the household, worrying over finances and planning ahead, cancer plunged her into a state of agonizing uncertainty.

Barb had always been strong for her daughters, and now she needed their strength to support her. She wasn't used to relying on others for help, trusting that when she was flying without a parachute there would be something or someone underneath to support her. She had been working two part-time jobs to keep money coming in, and she had no idea how the family would make it through the four months of recovery that stretched ahead. Cancer took away Barb's sense of control, but through the loss she found a deep inner strength that enabled her to feel safe in uncertainty.

> Out of my breast cancer experience I have gained a better understanding, respect and love of myself and now recognize that I have the strength to deal with whatever comes my way. I had watched others go through crises and wondered how I would react to an unexpected, negative experience in my life. I discovered an inner strength that gave me emotional energy to take each step as it came.
>
> I have been riding my benevolent dragon since my diagnosis and have learned to enjoy or at least to learn from every minute of the ride. Riding this dragon has enabled me to accept my life and all the changes it has brought and will continue to bring. I understand there is no script for life.

Barb learned to live in the moment and take each event as it came. Life became a more spontaneous and playful event.

The women's stories suggest that the two main qualities of one who rides the dragon are the ability to trust one's own nature and to trust the intelligence of life. These qualities – honed through the experience of uncertainty and exposure to death – are the very qualities that make it possible to truly live.

Fran kept a journal through her cancer and reflected deeply on the strength that emerges when all your hopes and expectations for the future are suddenly stripped away. Serious illness like cancer forces people to dig deep within to find out who they are, what they believe and why they are here. Said Fran:

> Cancer prompts us to dig to the very core of our being, our spirit, to touch the strength and true beauty that makes us persons and takes us up and through life and possibly on to the next. This is the strength we need. I think that in terms of all things working to the good, cancer can be that crazy backward gift that makes you dig to the core. It produces strength and gifts that you didn't know you had, and now you can claim them, and when you do, they glow.

Akky too spent time reflecting on the nature of the inner strength that she acquired through her journey with cancer, and what it means to have strength.

> I never thought of myself as having strength. I thought strong meant physically strong, muscular and having stamina. Strong meant being able to run long distances and being fast. Strong meant lifting and moving heavy things. I thought my mother was emotionally strong because she has a dominating personality and an ability to control others. I always thought strength was getting your own way through dominating others.
>
> Now I know that strength means feeling secure enough to take risks and try new things. After going through cancer, I feel I can handle other crises and setbacks as well. I can ask for

help and support and I can give it back. Strength also means being able to say no.

When I look at the strength in me and the strong women I know, I think strength is being able to sort out what you want, and live your life the way you want. It means knowing yourself and having the courage to stick up for yourself without dominating or manipulating others. It has nothing to do with physical strength or being a bully or controlling. It comes from within.

At the same time, the women acquired an ability to trust the supportive nature of the world around them. Each in her own way found that when she was hanging in mid-air, she came into contact with an almost magical web of love and assistance. Pamela, who felt abandoned and alone through her cancer, experienced that love and support when she joined the Vancouver dragon boating team. She vividly remembers the day she was steering the boat and things suddenly went wrong.

 One evening at practice, the wind and a strong current (tide change) caused me to lose control of the boat. I started to turn quickly – terrified of crashing. When I realized I was out of control, I yelled, "Help!" My team reacted instantly and stopped the boat immediately. I felt very relieved and thankful. I'm not used to asking for help, so to get it so easily was great! The experience left me feeling shaky and very humbled, however. I knew I had to get right back on my horse to get my confidence back.

The vote of confidence from my team is a good example of the strength dragon boating gives to me. The new friends who love and validate me are my new family. There is strength in numbers and a collective strength I feel in the group. I have a more solid sense of security. It's so good to have a safety net.

Fran found that web of support in the hospital when she was recovering. It came from family, friends and strangers; even the light in the room seemed infused with golden warmth and intelligent kindness.

🍃 This cancer journey was eased by the compassion and encouragement of friends and family – cards, flowers, letters. Friends prayed and promised that all would be well. They said I would be surrounded by a "golden light" during surgery. On awakening from surgery, the voice of staff kept saying, "Open your eyes, look at the *golden* roses. They are so beautiful." How often do flowers arrive at the bedside to greet you on your return from surgery? Those roses assured me that the "golden light" of protection had indeed surrounded me when I was not conscious.

Prayerful friends assured me that "guardian angels" would protect me. My primary nurse during all of the days of hospitalization wore six angel pins on her uniform! What an affirmation!

Recovery from surgery was almost buoyant in a hospital room with a glorious western view, with flowers in the foreground, including an entire rose bush. Flowers and cards said *Get Well, Happy Birthday* (60th!) and *Happy Mother's Day*. (The family got off easy... three wishes for the price of one!) Lovely May weather helped to keep the flooding Red River from doing even further harm and allowed me to recuperate. It was time to get down to our lovely camp on Lake of the Woods, another healing environment. Life was beginning again to flow fully, through the healing forces of the spirit expressed in family, friends, physicians and nature.

Barb Mitchell, who was so worried about the loss of control, found that there was more strength and support in her family and friends than she had ever imagined.

🌿 I was overwhelmed by the support my daughters and I received once people knew I had breast cancer. I really appreciated the human connection – and that ranged from shared tears, funny cards, beautiful cards and flowers to slow walks on the seawall. While we didn't go around shouting my diagnosis from the rooftops, we were honest with people when they asked how we were. The girls relied on their friends for support and I was relieved they had so many close friends to share this emotional rollercoaster with. I was amazed by these teenagers' capacity for compassion and concern. We were open about what I was going through, and everyone we knew seemed to know just how much sympathy, humor and even food we needed. Mothers of my daughters' friends dropped off casseroles and goodies, and I received enough books to keep me busy until I went back to work. Knowing that all these wonderful people cared helped more than they could ever imagine.

With inner strength and trust in the supportive nature of the world around them, the survivors entered a new realm. They went from being land dwellers, concerned about security and certainty, to air dwellers, living in a dynamic, spontaneous and spiritual realm. The world no longer seemed to be a hostile place that they needed to control or defend themselves against. It was full of friendship, support and guidance from within and without. They began to ride the dragon as they accepted their new lives and the very real possibility that in cooperation with their dragons they might be led to the fulfillment of their deepest wishes. As the poet Rainer Maria Rilke once wrote, "Perhaps all the dragons of our lives are princesses who are only waiting to see us once beautiful and brave. Perhaps everything terrible is in its deepest being something helpless that wants help from us."

New Dimensions

Through their ordeal with cancer, the survivors were taken to new places. Having faced the dragon, wrestled with it and ultimately come to ride it, new dimensions of life opened up to them. In this new realm there were no territories that were denied or off limits, no discussions they couldn't have, no dark places they couldn't go. They were living in a new way, with a rejuvenated sense of purpose and direction. New creativity, new opportunities, new friendships, were possible.

Akky was able to travel far beyond the perimeters of her once narrow and contained life. Before her cancer she had worked in a small room in a private school, hidden from view and afraid to take risks. After, she flew an airplane and steered a dragon boat. She stood up in the boat, completely exposed, and led her teammates through race after race, confident that she could steer through whatever wind and weather came her way. Riding her dragon, Akky's horizons expanded while at the same time she felt a new sense of belonging in the world.

🍃 This dragon is taking me to new places I only dreamed of going to. Not as an outsider, as a visitor or a tourist, but as one who belongs here. I now can see the wonders of nature, the wilderness, gentle pastoral lands, and works of beauty of man-made structures and the bustle of cities and how all these things interconnect. People are all part of it, including me. The dragon can fly high above it all and yet I feel closer to it than ever. Below, the human drama unfolds, with so many stories to be told. The world never looks the same through cloud, mist or clear air. The lighting is as varied in color and intensity as the minutes in a day. The rays of light shining through holes in the cloud seem like beacons from heaven, rays of light, hope, and the promise of things to come.

Brenda Tierney expressed the same feeling of belonging when she started hiking. Having found pathways through cancer, she now climbed to the top of mountains.

🌿 Since having cancer, I have become a hiker. One of my favorite places is on the top of one of the mountains I hike. The hike is always worth the exhaustion because of the beauty that waits at the top. The beauty lifts my spirit and feeds my soul. I feel part of the cosmos – all that has been and all that is.

Just as the dragon took the survivors outward, expanding their ability to move, travel and relate to the world, it also deepened their appreciation of life – slowed them down and enabled them to savor each moment. Creativity flourished as the survivors spent time with their children or took time to watch the birds, the clouds, the rain and the flowers. Bernice found herself enchanted by the tiniest wonders of the physical world and spent hours painting what she observed.

🌿 I've gotten a lot more serious about my painting, mainly because I didn't give myself the time before. Now I make the time. The year of my diagnosis, I think I did between 150 and 200 paintings, mainly of plants and flowers. I like to do the scientific-looking things, so you feel like you can pick a berry off the page.

Sometimes I get really, really serious about a tiny thing and I'll spend a whole hour just sketching it. And other times I just let loose.

I'll tell you a funny thing. I started painting a hazelnut bush one day when my husband and I were camping. Then a little ladybug crawled up on one of the leaves, and I thought, *Oh great, I'm going to paint the ladybug.* So I painted it on the leaf with the shadow and everything. Later on, one of the other campers came up and said, "Oh, can I see what you're doing?" Then she reached over and she tried to flick the ladybug off the picture. She said, "There's a bug on your painting!"

The dragon took the survivors deep into the heart of the world, opening up their compassion, their sensitivity, their capacity to touch and be touched. Before their cancer, many didn't know how to face people who were sick and suffering, let alone comfort them. But having gone through it themselves, they were able to listen open-heartedly to the pain, fear, sorrow and suffering of others. As Akky said:

> The dragon has taken me to parts of myself I didn't know were there. It has awakened a side of me that I didn't know existed. I can encourage and comfort others, as well as be comforted and encouraged by others. It has taken me to a world of illness and mutilated bodies, pain and suffering, that I would have avoided at all costs. Now I see the courage there. I am comfortable with women, myself included, who dress and undress with no thought of their deformity. No one notices after a while. It is part of life, part of the battle to survive, war wounds. Some are even proud to show their wounds and compare themselves to Amazons. It is sometimes the source of great humor. I no longer buy clothes to hide my scars. This is the way we are.

Through their journeys, the women found themselves more accepting of their humanity. They described themselves shedding worries, defenses, procrastinations, inhibitions and doubts. The dragon was taking them to a place of ever-expanding, ever-deepening reality, making it possible for them to be truly present for every moment of life. As Julie Davey-Prior said:

🔥 I think my dragon is helping me to always be authentic. I don't want to be something I'm not. My dragon is helping me to be more and more real and true to myself – to honor all my emotions and feel everything I need to feel.

I don't hide myself. If I start crying, then that's absolutely okay by me. I'm not prepared to take care of other people in terms of my emotions. They are what they are.

🔥 Flying high, no longer alone,
in the company of great heroes,
great warriors.
Women strong and free,
touching the sky.
The fierce dragon who reared its head
    from the dungeon of death
to destroy and devour me,
guarding its great secrets,
is now taking me places I never dreamed of
The messenger of death, destruction and loss,
    transformed to gentle vapor,
clouds in the sky
Now helping me fly high
Friends, family, children
nurturing, energizing, transforming,
opening doors
to places I never dreamed of,

removing unseen barriers
Barriers, walls of fear and ignorance,
   unseeing eyes, distrust,
all dissolving in the mist.
A Phoenix risen from the ashes of death.
The dragon is tamed, transformed,
like the butterfly out of its cocoon
Our ally, our friend, and so it transforms us,
It is us, we are the dragon.
A dragon that has control, direction,
   and purpose,
Light, hope, choices, power, strength
Fire
Water
Sky
Earth
Life
Energy
  – *Akky Mansikka*

The dragon-riding image in both Akky's and Qu Yuan's poems is not unlike the image of the charioteer which can be found in mythologies around the world. In *A Dictionary of Symbols*, J.E. Cirlot refers to the charioteer as a symbol of one who has harnessed himself or herself in the service of the soul. Those who ride the dragon have found a way to cooperate with the limits and necessities of fate, including losses and disappointments. Like the rider of a horse, they have opted not to "break" the beast, according to their will, but to develop a relationship of trust, honoring and respecting life's conditions while, at the same time, holding faith with their mission and goals.

As Rollo May said in *Freedom and Destiny*, when we acknowledge our limits and our losses, we engage our destiny. We do not always have control over the conditions of fate, and yet we do have what May called the "essential freedom" to choose what sort of position to take. Those who face the real conditions of their existence wrestle with their dragons until they find their own position. Once they see the new possibilities and directions suggested by the very limits they struggled against, they begin to ride the dragon, gaining power and momentum through their cooperation with the forces of life, just as the sailor or the pilot meets the wind, sea and stars.

How do we know when to impose our will and when to surrender to the larger forces at work and be carried to an unforeseen place? It seems that dragon riding is a very old art. In the ancient voice of Hadrian (quoted in Rollo May's book), who had also emerged from illness: "I was better, but in order to contrive with my body, to impose my wishes upon it or to cede prudently to its will, I devoted as much art as I had formerly employed in regulating and enlarging my world, in building the being who I am, and in embellishing my life." One thing is certain: to ride the dragon we must not be afraid to fly wherever we are called to go – even into the valley of the shadow of death.

The Dragon's Realm

The Dragon speaks:

*"... I am the old dragon found everywhere on the globe of the earth,
father and mother, young and old, very strong and very weak, death
and resurrection, visible and invisible, hard and soft; I descend into
the earth and ascend to the heavens, I am the highest and the lowest,
the lightest and the heaviest; often the order of nature is reversed in
me, as regards color, number, weight and measure; I contain the light
of nature; I am dark and light; I come forth from heaven and earth;
I am known and yet do not exist at all; by virtue of the sun's rays all
colors shine in me, and all metals."*

The realm of the dragon is not a binary realm of "either/or," it is
always "both." The Chinese celebrated the play of opposites, the
yin and the yang, and they believed the dynamic tension between
them generated the wonderful, multi-faceted world. They symbolized the paradoxical nature of reality in the t'ai chi, a circle bisected
by an S, with light on one side and dark on the other. There is a spot
of light in the darkness and a spot of darkness in the light, suggest-
ing that we not forget the opposite in either sphere. The one who
journeys through the night is reminded of the day, and the one who
revels in the day is reminded of the night. In this way, as old King
Hrothgar suggested, the guardian of the soul remains awake.

The Shadows of Death

To ride the dragon, the survivors had to be willing to expose themselves to the constant reality of death. Brenda Welsh put it this way:

> 🌿 I would say that dragon boating has taken me to a place where death stares you in the face. Several women have died and several have had recurrences. I feel at times that death hovers over us. It swarms around and just randomly strikes. At times I wonder who will be next. I don't like thinking about this, but it is a reality.

Barb Chomski almost quit dragon boating because she found it so difficult to lose friends on the team.

> 🌿 The first time it happened was the worst. We had gone to Montreal by bus, and I was sitting with Julie Davey-Prior and we really got to know one another. One of our other teammates, Barbara, was with us too. We had a great time in Montreal, and then Barbara and her husband decided to stay on in Quebec, sightseeing and whatnot, and we went home. A few days later we got a phone call that Barb had died in Montreal.
>
> She died of leukemia. Her blood count was low, maybe due to the chemo. She had been really tired, and she and her husband ended up going to hospital in Montreal. That's where she died. We were shocked. She *raced* with us! As a matter of fact, when we first heard the news, we thought she had died in a car accident.
>
> So then there was the funeral and, boy, we got to see what a dragon boat meant to her. All the dragon boat stuff was laid out by her casket.

Then our team got together at Eleanor Nielsen's house, and we talked about Barb. Then one of our members, Maria, started to cry. Later on, over tea, Maria said she was afraid her cancer had come back. It had. Not long after, Maria passed away and we went to her funeral. Then, at Maria's funeral, when we were walking away from the gravesite, another teammate, Georgie, said, "I'm afraid I'll be next." She was. Five months later, Georgie died.

After the loss of Maria, Barb couldn't bring herself to return to the boat, and she felt very troubled until she came to a decision.

🍂 After Barb died, I thought, *Holy smokes.* I couldn't make the next practice. I couldn't face seeing that spot where she used to sit. And then I talked to my brother-in-law up at the cottage. I said, "I don't know how I can return."

He asked me, "How can you put your cancer behind you if you're faced with death all the time?"

I realized, *I'm never going to put this behind me. It's part of who I am.*

STRUGGLING WITH OPPOSITES

The survivors live in a realm where opposites are expressed everywhere. The dragon boat itself contains a contradiction – it is both a vessel of hope and a grim reminder of death. It is powered by women who are weak and strong, sick and well, old and young. The very sport of dragon boating for women with breast cancer originated out of a contradictory response to recovery. While conventional medicine prescribed rest, Dr. Don McKenzie in Vancouver decided to offer women a completely different solution. In 1996, when he began the first dragon boating team, he challenged survivors to build strength from the very muscles they had lost.

The breast cancer teams are open to women in all stages of recovery; there is no criteria for fitness, performance or age. While other boats may be loaded with the most able and developed bodies, the women in pink are a motley group that includes every age, size, shape and physical condition. They train as hard as the other dragon boaters, but the context in which they race is completely different.

When Marjorie joined the Toronto team at the age of 73, she found that she was the eldest among the team members. At first she was reluctant to join.

> When I was asked, "Are you going to join the team?" I said, "Oh gosh, no! I'm too old," and my friend said, "Nonsense! How old are you?" I said, "I'm 73!" and she said, "They'll love you, just go, just go."
>
> So I went, and that first year was great fun. I was a rarity. I must have been 30 years older than anyone else. I felt very welcome and people took great pride in saying, "One of our members is 73." Several people at a coffee meeting with our sponsor said, "You're amazing! How wonderful that you can do that. I think that's great."

Marjorie's presence on the team gave confidence and encouragement to newcomers who were in doubt about their ability to join. She made it possible for many to get on board who might not have done so otherwise.

> When people tell me, "I'd really like to paddle, but I don't know if I can do it; I'm not that strong," I've said, "Look, if I can do it, you can too!"

Many survivors were heartened by the variety of fitness levels and ages that they encountered on the team. They came to their first practice feeling nervous, vulnerable, weakened by chemotherapy and radiation, and were relieved to be warmly greeted by teammates who understood their anxiety. Marian was one of many women who started out fragile and discouraged, and was carried to strength by her teammates' compassion and encouragement.

🖊 The toughest moments were the first few on-the-water practices. Because I had been recovering from treatment and surgery, I had had no time to train. The first few times on the water were really hard – my back ached, my arms ached and I simply couldn't keep up with the rest of the boat. I felt so discouraged and wondered how in the world I was ever going to do this. Then my seatmate leaned over and said, "That's okay. You can do this. If you get tired, just lily dip for a few strokes until you can paddle again. Don't worry about it." It was just what I needed to hear. I picked up my paddle and felt very fortunate to be part of this team.

For Marian and many others, the most important role of the survivors' dragon boat team is to provide a "support group" for women who are recovering, and a means of helping them back to strength in body and spirit. Said Marian of the Calgary team Sistership:

🖊 Sistership is much more than just a dragon boat racing team. Sistership is a support group, and its members have a special bond based on a shared experience. We remember those who have lost their battle with cancer and the organization is actively involved in breast cancer fundraising and awareness. I am so proud to have been a member of this team, to know these women and be a part of their special mission.

At the same time there are strong, competitive women on the

team who, like Irene Hogendoorn, want to compete on a level playing field with other teams, and win races at the international level.

> ❦ My most incredible moment in dragon boating was when I was picked to represent Canada at the European championships in Sweden. I, along with four other members of Dragons Abreast, proved to ourselves and others that cancer survivors can compete with everyone on a level playing field if the motivation is there. Through hard work, determination and belief in the dragon's spirit, any success is achievable.
>
> Paddling had never been so easy, so rewarding, so effortless … so magical!

Team members like Irene give strength and spirit to the team as well as something to emulate. At the same time, the fact that breast cancer teams are made up of women of all ages and strengths challenges the teams in a unique way. They're not the kind of teams that are purely designed to win races, and yet they're in a competitive sport where the goal is to win. Consequently, a certain tension exists between the desire to win and the desire to support, and it intensifies when the team is in the heat of competition. The question becomes, "Who do we put on the boat? Do we fill it with the strong and experienced, or do we fill it with the whole spectrum of breast cancer survivors?" If only powerful paddlers are selected for their ability to win, then other members of the team feel excluded and the effects on the team can be divisive and even traumatizing. Barb Mitchell expressed the tension she felt when this occurred on her team.

> ❦ The only time I felt unsure and negative was during my first year, when it seemed I might not paddle in the Breast Cancer Challenge Race at the Alcan Festival in Vancouver. The team I was on was focused on winning the challenge,

and the idea of going with the "best" paddlers for that race was being considered. At that moment, all my insecurities came out and I realized how badly I wanted to be "one of the best."

To Barb's relief, the team decided to include all the paddlers in the challenge race, and that decision rallied all the available strength of the paddlers – weak and strong. It had a huge impact on the health of the team spirit.

🌿 I will never forget the thrill of marshaling with over 200 other breast cancer survivors for that race. As we lined up at the start line I had to remind myself to breathe and found it hard to resist the urge to sit back and relish the moment. The time between the "paddles up" call and the gun going off seemed to take forever. I barely remember the actual race as I followed the commands of our drummer and concentrated on getting the most from myself and my paddle. We won that race, and I can't say I didn't enjoy that experience. I guess I'm more competitive than I thought I was. The most important aspect of that first festival was the realization of how huge an impact our group had on everyone at the festival. I was so proud to be part of this incredible group and to wallow in their support and positive energy. In the beginning I drew from that well of support but am now feeling the need to give back and replenish the stockpile of goodwill this group creates. I do this knowing that I may have to draw from that well again in the future.

Reconciling Opposites

As survivors of breast cancer, the women's rallying cry is, "We're all in the same boat!" They share a common mission: to show others who are weakened by the struggle with cancer that there is life after the disease. In the back of their minds they are conscious of the people on shore who, like the poet Qu Yuan, may be saved by the hope they generate. As Bernice said:

> Getting our mission statement out there, that's what counts to us. I could care less if I was the last person off the last boat, as long as I was there and I was able to say to somebody standing on the shore, "You know, if you've got a loved one sitting at home who feels that they can't do anything, tell them to come and watch, tell them about us, tell them to go talk to doctors and people in groups, and find out that, yes, you can do other things, you'll live, but you have to want to!" I really firmly believe that if you don't want to live, you can easily let yourself go.

Because they are united in this profound way – bound by the higher principle of inclusion – their challenge is literally to pull together when the gap between them widens. Those who choose to race with both the stronger and weaker paddlers on board are compelled to harmonize their differences. From her drummer's perch at the head of the dragon, Julie Davey-Prior acts as a conductor, attuned to the feelings of all the paddlers as they race. She can see when someone is falling behind.

> If I see someone struggling to keep up I might say something to help that person, to give them a little more energy or a little more belief. I might tell them, "You can do it, you can,

you've got more. This is our race!" And sometimes that person is able to regroup and come back again.

At times, in order to allow one person to regroup, Julie will slow the pace of the whole boat. This action demands a sacrifice from the strong paddlers, especially the pacers up front, whose instinct is to power through when they see the boats inching ahead of them in the race. But all eyes are focused on the drummer, and everyone, including the pacers, completely trusts her. When Julie slows the boat down, the powerful paddlers surrender a little of their ferocity, and the women who are flagging get a little room to recover. They dig deep. Everyone comes into sync, and a marvelous power is with them. Their strokes may be slower, but they have force. Said Julie:

> 🌿 Once I slow them down and they're all reaching together, you feel this power. You find that two plus two is a lot greater than four. The power when they're in sync is phenomenal. When I ask them for more, it feels like they can give more.
>
> I tell them: "I don't care how you place, but you're going to *look good!*"

When they come into this power, the dragon is present; the boat lifts off and flies across the water. From her position in the stern, Akky described what the takeoff feels like.

> 🌿 When the boat is moving fast and the women are paddling in sync, I can feel the boat lift out of the water and ride high. It is as if the spray from the paddles and the wake it has created transform into wings, giving flight to the boat. I am there giving direction, calculating the heading, compensating for wind and currents, and seeing our final destination. It is as exhilarating as a flight in the air.

Dragon boaters live for the moment when the "many become one" – when the boat, like a wingless dragon, seems to fly past time. Some women remembered crossing the finish line, looking back over their shoulders and wondering, "How did we *get* here?"

Because the survivors race with a mission that goes beyond winning, they are compelled to find the power that comes from inclusion. It is deeply felt and brings them together as one, but it may not win races. Yet they are racing to win. How can they have both? Shouldn't they choose one or the other? It seems like a paradox; yet, as Fran commented, the paradox is not to be resisted.

> Yes, it's a conflict. Dragon boat racing is not just taking a boat on the river for a paddle. We are in a competitive sport. As long as one is in a competitive sport, one has to acknowledge there is a win and lose. There is room for both. If we just want to go for a paddle in a river, that's really good. But if one wants to enter a competition, then acknowledge that indeed it is one. But on the flip side of the coin, and simultaneously, one is a winner the moment one enters the club. (That's the good part about being human – you can live in three dimensions at once. It's a paradox, but it's an interesting truth!)

It is tough to live in the realm of the dragon. You have to be able to contain opposites, to live with the tension between them and use that tension for creative purposes. In Asia and East India, people have long understood that the conflict between opposites is the very generator of life and growth. Rational or not, that's the way life *is*. Eventually, all the survivors come to embrace the paradox that while they are in the race to win, they have already won, just by being there. As Dr. McKenzie said, "We have a phrase that accurately describes our race experiences: *We seldom place, but we always win.*" It is enough to have survived, to be alive, let alone to participate in such a vibrant, energetic event. In Marjorie's words:

❧ Dragon boating is not something everybody can do, even well people. Lots of people have said to me, "I don't know how you do it; I couldn't do that." Paddling is hard work. It's not easy to get 22 people in a heavy dragon boat and get it to go fast. That takes a while, but with practice we become pretty good at it, and our teams do win races. It's exciting to win, but it's never mattered to me, win or lose. I do my best, and more than that I cannot do, and nobody can. If we win, that's great, and if we lose, we tried!

Indeed, the real winning is just being there. I have a little card on my fridge. It's a picture of a dragon boat in the path of the sun, and it says, "I am a winner," and I feel I am. I never let it get to me. I was determined right from my surgery on that I was going to be perfectly normal, and live, thank you. And I am determined that I shall continue to do so, God willing. I'm 77 now.

The Pink Flower Ceremony

For the survivors, the contradictions of winning and losing, living and dying, are played out in every dragon boat race. They fight with all their will and determination to win, and at the end of the race they toss their pink flowers into the water, remembering those who have lost the battle for life. Barb Mitchell described what it is like to be part of the ceremony:

❧ One of the most emotionally charged aspects of breast cancer survivors paddling has become the symbolic throwing of pink flowers in memory of someone who has died of breast cancer or is going through a recurrence. This is traditionally done at the end of a Breast Cancer Challenge race. In the moment the flowers are being tossed into the water, the paddlers are lost in their own memories of the friends they have lost to breast cancer, and friends who are battling it at the time. The moment is a very real reminder of how vulnerable we all are. We paddle back in, tired, saddened, but also filled with pride for our accomplishments and for the statement we have made.

One might wonder why the women don't simply focus on winning back their lives and slaying the dragon of breast cancer. Instead, they have chosen to create a ceremony at the end of the race that keeps their wounds open, their losses present. But as Evelyn said, "We never forget. We must never forget." With every new season, when the dragon boats are taken out of storage and "awakened" in the "dotting of the eye" ceremony, the women tone their bodies and open their hearts simultaneously, preparing to win and lose, to celebrate and mourn. Just as the race celebrates victory, health and life, the pink flower ceremony honors the reality of loss, sickness and death.

At the same time, there is a deeply healing aspect to the pink flower ceremony. It has helped many women come to peace. At first, Anita found it very difficult to be continually reminded of her losses through dragon boating, and she wrestled with her love of the sport and the upset it caused in her. She had not come to terms with the death of her dear friend Linda, whom she described as her "lifeline to sanity." She and Linda had met when they were both struggling with alcoholic spouses. Linda died of cancer at the age of 41, and when Anita's cancer was diagnosed at 49, her struggle with the senselessness of death intensified. She had not been able to let go "of the pain and personal grieving and the memory of loved ones gone." Then one day, while watching her pink flower drift, Anita came to peace.

🌿 When I tossed my flower into the ocean, my internal feelings were at war. Then as the carnation drifted with the tide, I felt that I was being cleansed and reassured. I don't really know why; it simply happened. The actual action of tossing the flower signified the casting away of unidentified fear, worry and pain that I'd been carrying with me for years, even before my diagnosis. A formerly unrecognized peace flowed into me.

The interminable struggle of facing death – others' and my own – ended in that moment.

I felt a huge surge of renewed determination run through me. The battle is never really over until death, but it didn't terrify me to keep fighting. I felt so peaceful, it was amazing.

When Barb Chomski returned to dragon boating after the loss of so many friends, she felt a deep sense of victory. She had faced the reality of death and would not look away. Moving through dark and fearful places, she realized, was part of what made her strong. She got back on the boat with a new understanding of the role that the dragon played in her life. By keeping her exposed to loss, the dragon helped her to grow ever more brave and open-hearted.

🌿 My "winning moment" in my journey with cancer and dragon boating was getting back in that boat after a teammate died. It was a winning moment because it was one more fear that I conquered. I can't speak for everyone, but I feel that the pink flower ceremony honors those women who have been taken away from us. It is a reminder that we are not to forget them, not ever. When I toss that carnation I am overwhelmed with emotion. I feel sadness all over again for the women I knew that have died, for the women that have been newly diagnosed, and for the many losses we all endure.

And I wonder, *Will I be one of these women who is represented as a pink carnation?*

Facing her fears and getting back on the boat made Barb even more appreciative of the women in her company and the ceremony that honored them.

> 🌿 I feel a very strong connection with all the women in the boats. When we link our boats together and toss the pink flowers, the need to win the race and compete is extinguished and we are *all* together against the same foe. In a very weird way I feel honored to be part of this special group, but the cost of membership is very high.

The pink flower ceremony is a vital part of the survivors' dragon boating experience, and some teams will go to great lengths to ensure that it is included. One summer at a dragon boating festival in Calgary, teams were prevented from tossing their flowers into the reservoir because it provides the city's water supply. But then something magical happened that allowed the Winnipeg team Chemo Savvy to perform their ritual. Cathy told the story:

> 🌿 Some mystery person delivered a beautiful bouquet of pink carnations to the race site. They arrived in our team's tent with a card that said, "Thank you for showing us how to live, love and laugh."
>
> Later in the evening, after the race, we took the bouquet and went down to the Elbow River. It was a beautiful scene; the rocks were reflecting the last bit of daylight as the sun set. We held hands and sang "The River," and then tossed our flowers into the water and watched. They glowed like neon as they traveled down what looked like a road of gold. We found out when we got home that one of our teammates, Val, had passed on the day before. I'm sure that we all tossed those flowers with Val on our minds.

In every race, the women play out the dramatic opposites of

winning and losing, living and dying. Family and friends, onlookers and other dragon boaters are drawn to the shore and touched by the flower ceremony. It is an expression of the power of ritual in modern life, and no witness walks away unmoved. The women in pink remind everyone that life is not just about winning, it is about losing too, and that even with their feverish determination to win the battle against breast cancer they are able to accept the inevitability of death. In a sense, by having the heart and the courage to make the sacrifice of opening their wounds again and again, the women are keeping alive that humility that the wise King Hrothgar instructed all dragon slayers to remember: everybody dies.

For Bernice, the most powerful of all the pink flower ceremonies occurred in June 1999, when dragon boaters from across the country gathered on the Fraser River in B.C.

💮 The Vancouver team Abreast in a Boat was host to teams from across Canada, from Nova Scotia to Victoria. We attended workshops together, we ate together and every team did a skit or sang a song. Then we gathered in the auditorium and Kathyrn Nicholson sang "The River." There were very few dry eyes in the hall.

The races took place for the next two days. In the final race for breast cancer survivors, we all raced together. Ten boats of survivors lined up – it was phenomenal. It gave me goosebumps just to be there. We raced, and after, we got our 10 boats together and we all converged into a V. We had 220 pink roses, and on the command of one person we threw all the roses into the water. Now it was raining out, not heavily, but you should have seen the number of people who had gathered to see that race. My sister was on the shore and she said there were people standing six feet deep; she was trying to get through to take pictures and people weren't moving.

After we tossed the roses, the boats started to go in

towards the dock, but instead of going in, there was a jam up, so all 10 of our boats were delayed near the dock. One of us (I think it was me) said, "There's Kathryn on the shore! Let's ask her if she'll sing her song to us." So we shouted, "Kathryn, can you sing the song?" And she said, "Well sure, I don't have my guitar with me, but I'll sing it, a capella." And so she stood there on the shore and sang "The River," the song written by Garth Brooks and Victoria Shaw.

She sang it without music, loud and beautiful. We all joined in on the chorus, and then the people on the shore caught on and they joined in. There we were together, on the water and on the shore, in the dribbling rain, all wet but not cold – we were warm, you know, our hearts were warm.

CARRYING ONE ANOTHER ALONG

The women in the dragon boat are helping one another – one's strength supports another's weakness, and in this way they carry one another along. They are all part of one glowing dragon, said Fran.

In dragon boating you are in the company of other women who offer their gifts, and their gifts become your gifts because you're part of the team, part of the whole, and the whole is greater than the parts. One becomes a part of an even bigger self, with all the strengths of the team. Each little strength is different. But one gets to claim a part of it and reflect and journey with it, which is awesome. The strength of the others carries you.

There is a dragon boater who is confined to a wheelchair and yet she came out in her wheelchair to cheer us on at the Winnipeg event. Should I be confined to a wheelchair because of metastases, I'm not going to sit at home. If she has the strength to do it, I will do it too. It meant so much to us as a team to have her out there cheering from the sidelines. Her strength became our strength. It added to our strength. There are many many many examples of women who give us courage, more or less dramatically. They've had a tough time and they've come through it and overcome it. So you know that you'll make a bigger effort. We're carrying one another through. It's uplifting; it's a wind, a breeze, the spirit that uplifts.

In the realm of the dragon, the women learn from one another what it means to live well and to die well, supporting one another through difficult experiences. Marian, who really struggled with the problem of how to live in the "shadow of the dragon," found her teachers and guides among her dragon boating friends.

    I remember once we were sitting around a table and everyone was telling their story. Two of the women were less than 40 when they were diagnosed. Both had been diagnosed in advanced Stage III and both had undergone stem cell recovery treatment. As we talked, these two women displayed courage, humor and dignity, while I felt like I was falling apart. We laughed about Genevieve standing in the aisle of a grocery store and realizing that she had forgotten her prosthesis. We laughed about Michelle's kids decorating her bald head with magic markers. I was amazed that they could laugh and joke about their disease even at the height of their battle for their lives. They were vital, alive, positive and optimistic. Together, they gave me an important perspective on cancer. They taught me how to laugh again and they taught me much about living well in spite of cancer.

Ironically, those who are dying give light to the living, and the survivors cherish fond memories of their teammates' humor and vitality in the shadow of death. Bernice and the whole Chemo Savvy team in Winnipeg lost their dear friends Maggie and Val, who made a lasting impression on everyone. Said Bernice:

> Maggie and Val were so crazy, I'm telling you – funny! We could say anything to each other. Val was doing some photography for us and she would follow us around with that silly camera. I had stretchy bandages on my knees as preventive medicine and after a race I was bending down to undo them, and guess who was behind me pointing at my backside with the video camera? Val said, "That's going to be the end of the movie!"
>
> Maggie also stays with me. If I get into someone's car and I don't like their music, I just have to think of getting into her car. She loved country music, and she would say, "If you don't like my music, get out!" It makes me laugh over and over again. Val and Maggie will both be with me when I'm 85 years old. They are there with me for life.

Every time they toss their pink flowers into the water, the women are privately remembering moments with those who passed on, visiting with their spirits. Evelyn described those who had died as her "angel friends" and she felt their presence on the boat. In particular she remembered her friend Maria, who showed her how to be happy and healthy in the face of illness and death.

> All four women on our team who have passed away were special to me, but none more special than my friend Maria. Maria took a special liking to me, and I to her. I'm not really sure why, it's just one of those things that's unexplainable. We had a kind of mutual respect for one another, and we both knew that neither one would hurt the other. She was and still

is somewhat of a mystery to me. She was beautiful, talented and strong-willed. She knew every word to every song that you could think of. There are so many moments that made an impression on me, but none more than about two weeks before she died, and she wanted to go shopping. So off we went to Costco, and there she was strutting down all the aisles with her bald beautiful head and leather baseball cap, not giving a damn what anyone thought amid all the stares. I couldn't believe it. She was a force to be reckoned with. The very same day she stopped at one of her clients, to pick up a check, and even mentioned that her bald head just might help get her that check that had been owing to her for some time. Always the consummate saleswoman, that was Maria. But never a complaint. Maria never wanted anyone to feel sorry for her, and she never wanted anyone to suffer, least of all her children. Last but not least, Maria was a damn good paddler.

Awareness of "Angels"

"Death is the wisest counselor of life," wrote Stephen Larsen in *The Mythic Imagination*. To be aware of death as a companion looking over your shoulder is the mark of a true initiate. She who has returned to the world from the regions of death has the ability to be in both worlds, to act as a "special intermediary or emissary to the spirit realm."

As a result of the fact that the survivors are continually exposed to death and dying, they live in the constant presence of "angel friends," who are with them in daily life as well as on the water. When they throw their flowers into the water, the spirits draw close. This year, the Chemo Savvy team lost three teammates, and to honor them they included three white flowers among the pink ones. As Cathy said:

> ❦ It was very special to name them, and they were with us that day in the race. After we threw the flowers, the white flower for Val brushed against my paddle. It was very special to feel her there. I knew that she had contributed to our win that day.

And Cathy divulged a little secret about the magical racing power of breast cancer boats:

> ❦ It's reassuring for me to know that those women who became our friends and were taken from us are very much with us on those race days. I wouldn't want to let the race organizers in on this little secret, but I think come race day we have an advantage because of all the people we carry along with us in our boat. You can truly feel their power.

Sometimes the survivors were surprised at how their angel friends appeared in the race. Marianne's mother died in the spring of her first year of dragon boating, and Marianne was still mourning her loss. Her mother had helped her in so many ways through her cancer, and then succumbed to the disease herself. When Marianne entered her first race, she was filled with sadness that her mother had not lived to share her moment of triumph.

> ❦ The first year I entered dragon boating it was July and my mother had just passed away that April. As we were paddling down to the starting line a tear fell to my cheek and I kept thinking of her, wishing she could have been there to see me paddle in the boat. She had seen me at low times, and I wanted her to be able to see me at a time when I was strong, when I was a fighter. I could feel myself getting weaker and weepier,

afraid I was going to lose it. Then this yellow leaf appeared from nowhere and landed on my shoulder. This happened in July, when all the leaves were green! I knew then that my mother was there with me. Yellow was her favorite color. My tears dried and once again I felt very powerful and ready to race.

Not only on the boat but in life, the women understand how those who have passed on continue to touch and inspire the living. The border between the dimensions of life and death dissolves as the dead maintain a real connection with the living. Chantal's father passed on in 1986, but he did not leave her.

🍂 My father never talked much, but he was a wise man and gave me good advice. I talk to him once in a while. When I need his advice, he gives it to me with no fail. He is still here with me. Whenever I have had to make a decision and felt I had no answer within me, I would go outside, look at the stars and talk to him. Within a few days the answer would be so clear to me. It is hard to explain.

In the summer of 1999, I made a wish. I said: "Daddy, I wish I could celebrate Year 2000 with the man of my life. I am tired of searching and always wind up in a dead-end." So, in October I met someone. I said to myself, *Okay, this is it. My father is sending someone!*

No! After two weeks I realized that he was not for me. It would have been a great mistake. So, I thought, *Oh well, my father cannot grant me every wish and give me all the answers.* Then out of the blue, a man I had known for three years, since 1996 (when I was first diagnosed with cancer) came across my path, a man that I had respected all this time who had been right in front of my own eyes. At last I have true love in my life. I am in better shape physically and I feel I can accomplish anything! It's great to be alive, you know, and happy!

My father, he is always there for me, even from above.

Franci's greatest spirit friend has been her maternal grandmother, her "Baba Rae," who died of colon cancer in March 1982. She lived energetically up to the very moment she died – and beyond.

🍃 Baba Rae Sorokin came to Canada from the Russian Ukraine at 17, leaving some of her family behind. The experience could have traumatized this young woman, but her power of determination to make it brought her to Alberta, and to my grandfather. Rae Sorokin was not just my grandmother; she was one of my best friends. She would read all the girls' Tarot cards, and remind us as women to go with our hearts and our true feelings or we would never be happy. She told us to make the best of our situations – she believed that till her dying day. She never let go until she said her goodbyes in person to every grandchild – all 12.

The day she was dying, I remember sitting and having a conversation with her, and she was talking about life being for the living. I thought, *Baba, you're dying.* She was so alive, even when she was dying. She had so much strength and she was passing it on to me. That's what she was doing. She was giving her strength to me. It's been with me ever since.

Since she died, she has come to visit me. The first time it happened, I was living in Edmonton. She came to me and we had a conversation. My cousin will call me from time to time and say, "Baba just came in." A lot of my cousins have said that she has come to them through dreams.

The ancient philosopher Heraclitus once said, "When we are alive, our souls are dead and buried in us, but when we die, our souls come to life again and live." Those whose spirits have survived the unsurvivable provide the living with our greatest source of inspiration, courage and comfort. Their humor, courage and love repeatedly confirm the wisdom that the survivors have gathered from the dragon: never stop living, even in the face of death. In the shadow of the dragon, the light of the world shines brighter than ever. It is, as it was for Beowulf, a beacon on the shore.

In February 2001, members of the Toronto team Dragons Abreast attended many funerals. Julie Davey-Prior attended four in a row, and in addition to undergoing this series of sad events, Julie found out that her own cancer was "galloping again." Once again it had spread to her organs, and this time to her brain. But her position with death remained the same. She upheld life in the face of death; she had no enmity for the dragon even in its darkest aspect. She was the companion of death, and its opposite in the dance.

Once you're into the battle against cancer, you can't stop. I didn't want to live my life only fighting, because that's all I would do with my time. I'd be going all over the country into all these trials, trying everything. Every waking day would be consumed with killing this dragon.

And I know people who are engaged in that, and they're frantic. They're living their lives that way and forgetting about having lovely tender moments with their partners, or walking in the garden and saying, *Isn't it wonderful.*

It's very hard to live both roles, thinking life is wonderful and enjoying life and at the same time being in battle. I couldn't live the two roles, it isn't my nature.

I have accepted death. It's not up to me. I don't know when that really came to me, but it was really important. You know, when I first got this cancer, I ate right, I stopped eating sugar, I ate all organic, I went vegetarian, I did Essiac, I did the whole thing… and then I got it again. And I said, "What have I done wrong?"

You know, when you're in battle, you either win or you lose, and I lost. And so it was liberating to say, "You know, it's not about that. I'm going to eat well because I want to live well. I'm going to do the healing journey program and the support groups and the dragon boating because I want to enjoy life and live it in a healthy way. But I'm not doing this to kill the cancer, because that's not where I want to be." I had to get away from winning and losing.

Julie's position with death recalls the stand taken by the Greek Epicurus, who said: "I must die. I must be imprisoned. I must suffer exile. But must I die groaning? Must I whine as well? Can anyone hinder me from going into exile with a smile? The master threatens to chain me: what say you?"

Where the Dragon Flies

*The benevolent and wise dragons of Japan, Korea, China and East
India are all very fond of pearls, and in artwork they are often depicted
ascending and descending in the sky, making a path of light through
mists and shadows as they roll the pearly orbs across the sky. The sea
dragons are known to horde pearls in their underwater palaces, and all
the eastern dragons proudly bear the pearl under their chin or on their
forehead. The pearl has many meanings, but universally it is the jewel
that grants wishes, the long-sought "pearl of great price."*

FULFILLING WISHES

Like the sky dragons who pursued their pearls through mist and
shadow, the women expressed their deepest wishes when they
were asked where their dragons were carrying them.

For some, the "pearl of great price" was to find peace and equa-
nimity with the conflicts and losses that are an integral part of life.
Chantal imagined flying her dragon to the Orient, to a place of
serenity and self-realization.

> 🌿 We would be riding to Asia. I would learn all the secrets of
> the Asian people, their way of life, their fascinating culture.
> My dragon likes calmness, he likes warmth. He would take

me there because it is a warm part of the world, and also
because the dragon knows that if he were to bring me there,
I would never be the same again! Perhaps it has to do with
Buddhism. Maybe the one who meditates is more calm and
has a better chance of leading a healthy life – healthy in mind
and body.

Franci also soared on her dragon to a place of safety, peace and
shelter.

  My dragon would be taking me high above the clouds, to a
  very safe place. Above the pollution, smog. My dragon would
  take me to a tropical island, where I would be welcomed
  with open arms by the natives. All my family and friends
  would be there. It would be clean, the waters calm and clear.
  The weather would be perfect every day, and if it did rain,
  it would be a soft rain, just enough to water the vegetation.
  It would be my Shangri-La.

Brenda Welsh imagined flying her dragon to China to adopt her
"dragon baby," and she hoped that once her wish was fulfilled and
she had the baby in her arms, the dragon's role in her life would
come to an end.

  My dragon would retreat into the hills of China and only
  be remembered as an ancient myth. For me the dragon has
  come full circle. My destiny is taking me to China, where the
  mythology of dragon boating started. I see this journey as a
  way of putting the cancer behind me and moving on.

Bernice saw herself riding her dragon around the world on a
mission of hope.

  My dragon would be taking me to China, where dragon
  boat festivals originated. Amid the colorful palaces, flags,

kites and banners would be the great dragon replicas and
the dragon boats receiving their blessings before the next
race. Instead of paddling, I would be seated near my dragon's
head so I could whisper into his ear – "Go like the wind!"

Yes, my dragon would take me everywhere. My costume
would be pink and I'd carry armfuls of pink roses. As we traveled around the world, people would ask what our mission is,
and I'd repeat the mission statement of all dragon boat teams
such as ours. And in memory of every woman who has gone
before me, I'd scatter roses on the waters.

Julie Davey-Prior's "pearl of great price" was a return to the wonder she knew as a child. When she befriended her dragon, he transformed into a long-lost friend from childhood, a humorous green
dragon with sparkling iridescent scales that she named "Puff."
Julie's dragon was carrying her towards the state of total presence in
every moment of life.

 🌿 The journey I'm on is a spiritual experience. My dragon
 allows me to see moments and take those moments in. I slow
 my life down and take in the moments. I just take a deep
 breath and I say to myself, *Feel that moment. Hear it, taste it, feel*
 it, help me BE.

Julie was a child at camp when she first heard the song about Puff.

 🌿 The other kids had been talking about this magic dragon
 named Puff. I had never heard of him. The camp counselor's
 name was Andy. (I thought it was so cool that she had a boy's
 name.) She played the guitar and when she heard that I didn't
 know the song, she said, "I'll come in your tent and I'll sing
 you the song." Well, she played it for me, and I cried and cried
 and cried. I loved that dragon.

The song is about a close friendship between a boy and his dragon that comes to an end when the boy grows up and puts away his childhood toys.

> *A dragon lives forever, but not so little boys*
> *Painted wings and giants' rings make way for other toys*
> *One gray night it happened, Jackie Paper came no more*
> *And Puff that mighty dragon, he ceased his fearless roar.*

> *His head was bent in sorrow, green scales fell like rain*
> *Puff no longer went to play along the cherry lane.*
> *Without his lifelong friend, Puff could not be brave*
> *So, Puff that mighty dragon sadly slipped into his cave.*

When Julie considered what moved her so much about the song, she said:

> ❧ It was so hard to give up my childhood. I cried when I turned 13, I cried when I turned 16, because I didn't want to grow up. I just loved my childhood, and that song was about that time. So that was the only connection to a dragon I had; he was that little boy's friend. He took him to wonderful, magical places and he gave him confidence.
>
> Now I have him back.

Julie Dubuc's dragon was taking her out of the past and into the future. To appreciate fully where she and her dragon were at that moment, she painted a picture called *Riding the Dragon.*

> ❧ The image is of me riding on a very fierce-looking dragon through the night sky and leaving a wake in the clouds behind. The dragon and I are paused in the air looking over at the future. My dragon is taking me to new heights of self-growth and belief in myself, and I know now that I can soar as high as I want to go.

Marian's dragon was also taking her through the shadows of the past and into a future brightened by new confidence and appreciation.

🌿 My dragon is taking me to the future – to new adventures, to more self-discovery. I don't know what the future holds for me, but my experience with cancer has been a seminal event in my life. Everyone wonders how they will react in a moment of crisis. Will they be able to rise to the challenge? I am proud of myself for having met the test, for being a survivor. I feel very lucky to be alive and I'm thankful for all the fellow journeyers and supporters I have met along the road. Now it's time to move forward and live the life I've worked so hard to reclaim.

Coming Home

T.S. Eliot wrote in "Little Gidding":

> *We shall not cease from exploration*
> *And the end of all our exploring*
> *Will be to arrive where we started*
> *And know the place for the first time.*

Through their incredible journeys, the women were ultimately brought back home to the place where they began. And while the places had not changed, the women had. They had become like the sea dragons, suffused with appreciation. Their homes had become their palaces, deep sanctuaries where they gathered in all that was precious and dear.

After her cancer treatments finished in August 1997, Cathy discovered St. Vital Park. The park had always been a feature of her neighborhood, but she had never paid much attention to it. "I didn't see any value in it as a destination," she said. Then one morning, she and her dog stumbled upon the place that would become her sanctuary.

> ❦ It was a beautiful fall day, the leaves were crisp and on the ground beneath our feet. Early morning we walked down the secluded trails of St. Vital Park, just my dog Hector and I, with the odd squirrel or chipmunk peeking out from the underbrush. He didn't see them; otherwise he would have bolted into the bushes. We went winding through the trails, passing the Red River as we plodded through the park. I could smell smoke in the air from the farmers burning their fields, and there was the slightest hint of sugar beets from the nearby sugar factory.
>
> This was a place where I could be alone in my thoughts, with my dog by my side, and figure out ways to rebuild my strength for the future.

For Cathy, St. Vital Park was a dimension of her life that she had never known before. It afforded the opportunity for long walks and quiet contemplation – a chance to inhale and appreciate the passing moments of life. The park invited her into the depths of her own being, and yet, on the brink of discovery, she worried that she might lose that precious sanctuary.

> ❦ That fall I had great fear that I would not see the spring from those secluded trails. But I have since seen it three times. Now it's easier to believe that there will be many more fall walks in the park as beautiful as the one that first day.

Ultimately, as Cathy realized, the dragon's journey is an ever-deepening experience of home.

> ❦ Have dragon, will travel! However, I don't think I would go

very far on my mythical dragon. I have a great appreciation for where my life has taken me, and am deeply content with my place in life now. If I were to take my dragon for a spin, I don't think I would go farther than a cruise down the Red River, to a place that's familiar and comfortable for me. I would take my family and friends along for the journey; they could ride on the dragon's tail. We might stop for ice-cream along the way.

The pearl has many meanings around the world, but perhaps none is so universally compelling as the idea that it forms out of the hard grit of suffering. In fairy tale lore, the princess is sometimes depicted as one who weeps pearls, particularly if she is strong-hearted. In one story from the Grimm brothers' collection, "The Goose Girl at the Well," a true and loving daughter of the King is exiled by her father when she refuses to flatter him in exchange for a piece of his kingdom. In his rage, he divides the land between her two elder sisters and banishes her from the country. As the princess leaves and goes up the mountain, she weeps a path of pearls. She is taken in by a wise woman and for three years she tends the old woman's geese in a secluded mountain retreat. When her father finally repents and goes searching for her, he finds her in her mountain home. "My dear child," he laments, "I have given my kingdom away, what shall I give you?"

The wise woman says to the King: "I give her the tears she has wept on your account; they are precious pearls, finer than those that are found in the sea, and worth more than your whole kingdom."

Great wisdom, creativity, love and perspective come out of suffering. The dragon's pearl reminds us that while dragons may be terrible and ruthless combatants, they are connected with the fulfillment of our deepest wish, the thing that can bring us to peace and make the suffering all worthwhile.

Brenda's pearl was to hold her child in her arms at last. Marian's wish was to live fully the life she fought so hard to win. Julie Davey-Prior's pearl was to become as real and full of wonder as the child she once was. For many women the pearl expressed a future full of wonders they never would have dreamed possible had they not gone through the ordeal of cancer. And some, having fully embraced this contradictory world, voiced a wish for humanity, a wish for peace.

All together, the women are joined in their ultimate wish to give hope to others who are struggling with cancer. They shout to us through their pain and their tears and their paddle-spray: "We can't be defeated – even by death!" They show us what we are made of, that we are all dragon spirits capable of surviving grief, illness and death. They urge us to keep our dreams and wishes intact, wherever the journey takes us – to ride our dragons with courage, with a never-ending sense of mission and, above all, with an unwavering love. What the dragon holds or withholds, that is our treasure, our pearl of great price.

Once we have seen the women in pink out there on the water in their dragon boats, their voices are with us forever. They give us hope and comfort, the kind that will appease the fearful child who looks to his nurse for reassurance.

"Never turn away from a dragon," they whisper. "Our dragons make us *wise*."

Conclusion

Our dragons appear out of nowhere; their arrival is unforeseen. Whether they burst in aggressively or slip in secretively, they shatter plans and designs and throw lives into chaos. They have no respect for authority or worldly accomplishments or the imperative of peace in the kingdom. Their impact is senseless and utterly devastating. There is no monster in myth more frightening than the dragon. It is the ultimate predator, ravaging lives with a voracious even desperate appetite. In its deadly aspect it has been associated with ultimate evil, anarchy and destruction, and it is so powerful that it seems impossible, sometimes even ludicrous, to go up against it.

Our myths reflect us. They mirror what we know deep inside. And our myths tell us that a dragon can only be met by the most valiant spirit in the village – the one who is prepared to confront impossible odds. That dragon slayer dwells within each of us, in potential, awaiting the time when the dragon appears, as it inevitably will because life includes dragons. No kingdom is without them, it's just that we don't know when they will appear, because dragons come from that place below our awareness, that place of darkness and mystery that is beyond our control. No matter how far our kingdoms of consciousness reach, there are still dragons, and there will be dragons as long as there are unknowns.

What every dragon takes from us is the sense that we are in control. They strip us of our confidence that we can rely on our reality, on our bodies, even on our gods. If we are raising children, looking after others, pursuing our careers and goals, how is it that we can be so suddenly thrown off course? Did we know so little about ourselves, about our purpose?

Akky said that whenever she gets off course, her dragon brings her back on track, and I believe she tapped into something very true about dragons when she said that. They seem to hold the knowledge of all that is underneath us. We not only ride on the backs of dragons, we *live* on the backs of dragons. We never know when they will erupt like a mountain and begin to move us somewhere. We don't know where in the world we are in the first place; we just live with an illusion of where we are, made up of everything we have learned about the world from childhood. But under the sun and the moon and the stars, the truth is, we really don't know where we came from or where we are going.

But maybe our dragons know.

When I asked Julie Davey-Prior how she saw herself riding her dragon, and where she was headed, she said she was riding backwards. As the drummer, she has her back turned to the destination, her legs wrapped around the dragon's neck. Her relationship with her dragon had moved to a place of absolute trust; she was headed backwards into the unknown. We spoke in March 2001, and Julie died two months later, on May 28.

I am at a loss for words. I have never worked on such a moving book, and I am utterly humbled by the women's stories and the correspondence with powerful events in my own life. From the start of this book to its finish I have been witnessing my father wrestle with his dragon – through six months of chemotherapy and radiation followed by a radical surgery to remove his esophagus. Like the dragon women, he had to weigh the risks, figure out his best option and go into battle with his dragon. In the beginning he met his dragon weaponless, strength to strength. Then he went

through the next campaign, months of cancer treatment. He struggled to stay strong against the weakening effects of the drugs – and
he did, he came through it victorious. But when he went through
surgery, he met the biggest dragon of all. During the many days he
spent in ICU following his surgery, he was nearly overwhelmed by a
powerful "vision of hell" that depressed him so much he lost his
best sword: his humor. It took him many weeks to recover from
that drug-induced hallucination which brought him face to face
with the reptilian side of life. He was taken to a cold, dark, cruel
and indifferent place where he experienced the total absence of
love. But paradoxically, in its absence, he realized the value of love.
He experienced the compassion that joins us all together as one
heart, one being, connected to the earth, to the sun and the stars.
He returned to the world scarred and bewildered and beaten up,
but filled with new understanding, hope and meaning.

Our dragons seem to fly us right through the eye of our worlds.
They fly us through the absence, the emptiness, the loss that we try
to fill up or escape. My own dragon has been the baffling condition
of endometriosis, with its "blessings" of chronic pain and infertility.
I really met that dragon when I met the loss head on, when I finally
came to acknowledge that perhaps it was not in the cards that I
should have a child. I tried to adopt, and powerful circumstances
led me away from that direction, telling me in no uncertain terms
that that was not the way. I could have raged and struggled and rat-
tled the cage – and I did, for years, until I finally came to realize that
it was wasted energy. Maybe my will did not have all the answers.
Maybe there were deeper forces at work in my life that I would be
better to acknowledge and cooperate with. I did, finally. I said
goodbye to my dream baby, like Brenda did when she buried the
dream of birthing her own child, and I opened myself up to the
emptiness, and whatever possibility might be waiting in the
absence. By going through the void, I awakened seeds that were

able to germinate only when I gave up insisting on my own direction. I took that powerful feminine wish to nurture and I turned it to mothering in other ways. Then the dragon that had withheld so much from me turned around and began to show me worlds I could never have imagined possible. Like this one. Like this book.

As human beings we have so much weaponry, so much technology, to shield us from the forces of life and death. It is easy to become spellbound by the illusion that we know what we're doing, where we're going and what we want. Those who are good warriors and have many victories and few losses can become dangerously misguided, as King Hrothgar recognized. Warriors who are not also lovers end up alone, he told Beowulf, which is a sad fate considering that we will die anyway. Better to be the lover and ride the dragon backwards into the unknown, trusting that our losses will be our gains, that our kingdoms await....

In the old fairy tale "The Briar Rose," the princess was cursed to sleep for a hundred years. When the spell took hold, everything in the castle fell asleep with her – the people in the hall, the doves on the roof, the fire in the hearth. Then a thick hedge of thorns grew around the castle and it couldn't be penetrated, although that didn't stop hundreds of suitors from trying their luck to free the princess from her sleep. Those who stormed the castle died stuck on the thorns. But on the day the sentence ended, the princess awoke, the briars bloomed, the hedge opened and the prince who had been biding his time came through.

Some say he was riding a horse. But I wonder if it wasn't a dragon.

The Survivors

Each survivor wrote her story with the assistance of a Storytelling Guide. We began by asking the woman to describe the places from which they would be telling their stories. Their stories came from many different places, some real, some imaginative. We have included their storytelling places because each one reflects a beautiful quality of the storyteller herself.

Chantal Brunet

Chantal is 36 years old and lives in St-Léonard, Quebec, with her 9-year-old son, Francis, and her loving partner, Pierre, along with their new Shih Tzu puppy Fluffy. She was 30 years old when she was first diagnosed, and three years later she had a recurrence. For the last 18 years Chantal has been an executive assistant for VPs in large companies. During the writing of this book she decided to pursue her passion for writing and is now working on a certificate in Public Relations. When she has completed her course in the summer of 2002, she and Pierre plan to get married. Chantal is a member of the Montreal team Two Abreast, and dragon boating is her main hobby. She has dark brown hair and eyes, and a bright, beautiful smile. Her loved ones describe her as "a leader, passionate, very social, determined and funny."

She told her story from her cottage deep in the woods at Lac Viceroy in Quebec. Her grandfather bought the property when her father was eight years old, and there is "no phone, no TV, no pollution." She sat out on the dock, early in the morning, with a mug of coffee in hand. The lake was calm and clear; eagles soared overhead as she watched the last of the morning fog lift from the lake.

Marian Busch

Marian lives in Ottawa with her husband, Ken, and works as a business systems consultant. She was 36 when she was diagnosed in the summer of 1997. Marian has short brown hair, large brown eyes and a big smile. Her loved ones describe her as "a leader, indomitable, wise, driven and fun," and her husband adds "bold, tenacious, funny, smart and cute." Marian was living in Calgary when she was diagnosed, and she later joined the Calgary team Sistership. Her experience with cancer has had a profound impact on her personally and has helped her examine her life and her goals from an entirely new perspective.

Marian told her story from her sunroom, curled up in a big, comfy stuffed chair with a steaming cup of coffee. The room was warm, sunny and colorful, filled with flowers and plants – hibiscus, oleander, umbrella plants, African violets, variegated ivies, Christmas cactuses and begonias.

Barb Chomski

Barb lives in Toronto and is the mother of 26-year-old twin girls and a 19-year-old son. Barb's cancer was diagnosed on Halloween 1996, when she was 44. Over the course of her journey with cancer, Barb went back to school and received training as a social service worker specializing in work with the elderly. She has many interests, including a love of travel, dance and theater. She enjoys reading spiritual books and has a strong interest in ancient religions and mysticism. Her loved ones describe Barb as a "pillar of strength – compassionate, a little crazy, spontaneous and deeply loving."

Barb told her story from a meadow surrounded by trees on a clear summer day, when the air was sweet with the scent of grasses and wildflowers.

Evelyn Crofts

Evelyn lives in Newmarket, Ontario, with her husband and 16-year-old daughter. She has worked for the town of Newmarket for 20 years. She describes herself as "5 foot 2, eyes of blue," and her family adds that she is "strong, trustworthy, honest, kind and determined." In 1994, at the age of 40, she was diagnosed with metastatic cancer, and had a local recurrence in 2001. One of the 33 original members of the Toronto team Dragons Abreast, Evelyn enjoys decorating, refurbishing furniture, sewing and homemaking.

Evelyn told her story standing on a cliff in Nova Scotia, overlooking the ocean. From her vantage point "high but not too high," she could see an island inhabited only by seagulls and a lonely lighthouse. She could feel the fresh sea breeze on her cheeks, and smell the delightful aroma of wild rose bushes. Nearby there was a memorial for a sailor lost at sea. "This spot must have been his favorite too," she wrote. "No wonder, it's a little slice of heaven – and if I didn't know for sure that it was real, I would think that I was dreaming."

Julie Davey-Prior

Julie lived in Toronto with her husband, Rod, and their three-year-old yellow Labrador, Bennett. She was first diagnosed in 1995, when she was 38 years old, and then in February 1999 she learned that her cancer had metastasized. At the time of her first diagnosis Julie was teaching at Humber College in the Child and Youth Worker Program and going to university part-time towards her degree in Social Work. After her first bout with cancer Julie joined the Toronto team Dragons Abreast. When her cancer metastasized, she went from paddling to drumming. A cherished member of the team, Julie is described by her dragon boating friends as "energetic, enthusiastic, positive, fun-loving, engaging and full of laughter." Her cancer went into remission and then reappeared in the late winter of 2001.

Julie told her story while paddling in her canoe on "a beautiful cloud-dappled day. My dog Bennett was in the canoe with me. We paddled close to shore, taking in all the sights and smells of the forest. We came to our campsite – a wonderful home in the woods with a beautiful smooth outcrop of rock that reached into the lake and around the water grasses. I lit a small campfire and the circle became a sacred space."

Julie died on May 28, 2001, at the age of 44.

Julie Dubuc

Julie lives in Winnipeg with her partner, Denis, and she is the mother of five children, ranging from 4 to 22 years old. Julie was diagnosed in 1998, at the age of 45, shortly after the birth of her last child. At the time, she and Denis had just sold their Art Gallery and Tearoom in northern Ontario and moved to Winnipeg. Julie is a full-time visual artist, whose paintings reflect her philosophy of life. She belongs to the Winnipeg team Chemo Savvy, and her loved ones describe her as "motivated, passionate, generous and philosophical."

Julie told her story sitting by a stream near a fairytale cottage – an imaginary place that she found on one of her guided meditations. It is an old English cottage with a thatched roof, surrounded by beautiful gardens and a forest full of animals who often come to the clearing for food.

Anita Ewart

Anita lives in Prince George, B.C., with her husband. She has two grown children and a baby granddaughter whom she describes as the "precious gift I've lived long enough to see." Prior to being diagnosed with breast cancer at the age of 49, she worked as a mammographer and breast cancer educator. After her experience she pursued her love of writing and became a published freelance writer.

Her second diagnosis came 20 months later, and today she has been cancer-free for four years. She is a member of NorthBreast Passage, Canada's 22nd dragon boat team of breast cancer survivors. The team is an empowering force in her life and, in her words, "perhaps the most significant group I have had the privilege of joining. A poignant memory, forever."

Anita is medium height and small-boned, with silvery-gray hair. She smiles a lot and describes herself as "determined, happy, optimistic, motivated, involved, busy and content."

She told her story outside her home by the water, sitting in a warm breeze, with a flourishing garden nearby and homemade soup simmering on the stove.

Franci Finkelstein

Franci lives in Toronto and works for the airlines. She had just turned 38 when her cancer was diagnosed at the end of summer 1997, one week after her brother's wedding and a day before she was offered a new position with Canadian Airlines in Vancouver. It was a turning point in her life. A member of the Toronto team Dragons Abreast, Franci has a wonderful joie de vivre – a passion for life and living. If there is adventure to be had, Franci likes to take on the challenge, and she enjoys the beauty of the outdoors. Although petite, Franci is powerful – dark-haired, green-eyed, and full of energy and humor. Her loved ones describe her as "funny, good-natured, sensitive and loving."

Franci told her story sitting out on the front beach deck at "The Lake" at Mameo Beach in Alberta, where her family once had a cottage. It was early in the morning on a warm summer day, and she was holding a "lake-mug" of fresh coffee and waiting for her grandfather to return from his morning walk along the beach. She could hear birds singing and squirrels running about the evergreens as she watched the mist rise from the calm, silent lake.

Marjorie Greenwood

The oldest member of the Toronto team Dragons Abreast, Marjorie is 77 and lives in Toronto. Her husband died in December 2000. She has two daughters, five grandchildren, and two Burmese cats, Fred and Molly. Marjorie was diagnosed in 1992 at the age of 68, after which she became a Wellspring volunteer. Marjorie worked as an editorial assistant at the British *Vogue* magazine in the early 1940s. In 1944 she married a Canadian air force officer and they moved to Toronto the same year. In the 1950s and '60s, Marjorie was very active in theater and radio, and was twice awarded "Best Actress" honors at Hart House.

She told her story from the lodge at Deer Lake, where Wellspring holds a yearly retreat every September. She sat near the fireplace in the great room, looking out on the lake, where no motorboats are allowed and the water is still and smooth.

Irene Hogendoorn

Irene has been married to her husband, Ed, for 22 years and resides in Etobicoke, Ontario, with her teenage children, Kimberly and Adrian, and best friend Nika, the family German shepherd. Irene was diagnosed just after her 42nd birthday, and thanks to the love and kindness of her family, friends and doctors, she is happily paddling in any boat that will take her.

Dragons Abreast awakened Irene's spirit for the sport so much that she now paddles with the Canadian national team, competing in Sweden and, just recently, at the Worlds in Philadelphia. Irene has made dragon boaters out of her son Adrian and her best friend Rose. Hubby Ed has also been involved!

Irene told her story sitting on her deck with her dog beside her, looking out over the swimming pool and feeling grateful to be alive and well. As she reflected on her journey, she felt the warmth of the sun on her skin and heard the wind softly blowing through the trees.

Karen Kellner

Karen is married to her second husband, Terry, and they live in Toronto with her two teenage sons. Karen was diagnosed during the winter of 1995, when she was in her mid-forties. Karen describes herself as "5 foot 2, red-headed and feisty." She joked that if her friends were asked to say a few words about her, "I'm not sure I would want them printed!" She is nonetheless described as "loving and understanding, with a good sense of humor, non-judgmental and energetic."

She told her story from her home. "I know this sounds boring, but my healing really took place in the womb of my home, surrounded by my husband and children. We have a lovely, cozy tandem off our bedroom with windows on three sides. It faces our backyard and, beyond that, our local park. Nature and nurture – what more could I have asked for?"

Bernice A.M. Kwasnicki

Bernice lives in Winnipeg with her husband, and she is the mother of three grown daughters. When she was diagnosed at the age of 53, she had no family history of breast cancer. Bernice has many hobbies, which include music, writing and gardening, but her main interest is watercolor painting. In the summer months, when she is not dragon boating, she and her husband are traveling the country in their RV. A member of Winnipeg's team Chemo Savvy, Bernice is of medium build with gray-brown hair, and her daughters describe her as "sensitive, compassionate, generous, intelligent and artistic."

She told her story from her garden, amid peonies, tiger lilies, irises and many other wild and uncultivated plants. Her garden is home to many birds, rabbits and squirrels, and it is the place where four grandchildren are always hiding and rediscovering treasures.

Kaethe Lawn

Kaethe is married, lives in Victoria, B.C., and has a son and a daughter. Kaethe was born in Postdam, Germany, and she was a young child during World War II. In her words, she is one who "vividly remembers the brutalities that are the fate of the conquered." Kaethe came to Canada in her early twenties and lived in Montreal for 35 years. She was in her early forties when she was diagnosed with breast cancer, over twenty years ago.

Now a resident of Victoria, Kaethe paddles with the Victoria team Island Breaststrokers and she greatly enjoys not only the rigors and many challenges of this sport but also the spirited company of her fellow paddlers. Being very fond of the sea, she also kayaks and is a crew member of an outrigger canoe during the winter months.

Kaethe describes herself as "a typical dragon boat paddler: straggly hair from sun, wind and salt water, my hips just narrow enough to be wedged into the seat, permanent calluses on that part of my body that comes in contact with the two-by-fours (bravely referred to as benches by some), hands ruined beyond repair from prolonged immersion in ice-cold water, hunched shoulders to ease sore shoulders, two pronounced vertical lines between the eyebrows due to focusing in the boat!" She says her personality matches the boat: she is "quite stable, reliable, fast-moving given the right circumstances, some scratches here and there…can be swamped but will not sink… at times found gently rocking near the dock."

Kaethe told her story sitting at the computer, but in her mind she was on a piece of driftwood by the water's edge, her feet propped against a rock, overlooking the strait. "Seagulls were crying overhead, and a heron stood motionless, fishing."

Akky Mansikka

Akky lives in Toronto with her husband, Henry, and works as a special education teacher at a private school. She is the mother of three grown children. She was first diagnosed at the age of 46, and then again at 50, after which she had a double mastectomy followed by reconstructive surgery. Akky's friends and family describe her as "warm, loving, adventurous, hard-working and conscientious." After her breast cancer experience Akky took flying lessons, received a pilot's license, and then became a steersperson for the Toronto dragon boating team, Dragons Abreast.

She told her story from an imaginary beach on a tropical island that is teeming with life and provides a refuge from storms. "The whole scene is a feast for the eyes – the blue-green water, the white sand, the colorful tropical flowers and trees. You can only get to the place by slowly drifting there in a small boat."

Barb Mitchell

Barb lives in North Vancouver with two of her three daughters (the other daughter lives two blocks away). A former teacher, Barb now works as the head clerk at a screening mammography center and spends her spare time "puttering in my patio garden, cooking, walking with friends, skiing and, of course, paddling." She belongs to the Vancouver dragon boating team Abreast in a Boat. People who know Barb describe her as "compassionate, dedicated, sincere, reliable and giving." ("My God, I sound like a saint!")

Barb told her story from Lighthouse Park in West Vancouver, nestled into the rocks with a duvet and pillow. From this aerie she could see and feel the fresh and rejuvenating ocean.

Marianne Primeau

Marianne lives in Winnipeg with her husband, Don, and their little girl. Marianne was diagnosed when she was 39 years old, at a time when her husband had just settled into his new law firm and they were enjoying their three-year-old "miracle baby" after four miscarriages. Marianne is from a Ukrainian background. She has dark hair and dark eyes, and she describes herself as "quiet and shy (but I've come out of that a lot), very caring, a good listener. I have a sense of humor, I'm compassionate, and I'm a fighter." Marianne is the chairperson of the Winnipeg team Chemo Savvy and describes dragon boating as "adventure therapy."

Marianne told her story sitting on a "nice, quiet, white sandy beach by the sea, where the sand is warm – not hot – and feels soft, like icing sugar."

Cathy Prusak

Cathy is 38 years old and lives with her husband, Marc, in a lovely old Winnipeg neighborhood. Their pride and joy is their dog, Hector Suarez – "a schnauzer, German shepherd cross. We call him a 'Schnepherd.'" Cathy was 33 when she was diagnosed in November 1996. She describes herself as "5 foot 4, 130 pounds (give or take a few) and proud of my muscular dragon boat arms." Her husband says she is "good-natured, caring and smart as a whip," and her friends describe her as "dedicated, hard-working and adventurous."

Cathy told her story from St. Vital Park, a secluded place by the Red River that she discovered in the fall, shortly after she finished her cancer treatments.

Pamela Robbins

Pamela lives in Halfmoon Bay, B.C., in a house on the water's edge, with her cat and her dog. She was 51 when she was diagnosed, and it was not a shock as she had had precancer since 1975 and had undergone several lumpectomies. After her diagnosis in 1999, she had a bilateral mastectomy. In addition to paddling with the Vancouver team Abreast in a Boat, Pamela became a steersperson, which came naturally after years of steering canoes and sailboats. Steering was also a good way to regain some control in her life. She describes herself as a nature lover, a conservationist, an evolving woman and an explorer. Her friends describe Pamela as "spunky, resourceful, a good spirit, brave, an old soul…" An ex-teacher, she now works as a marriage commissioner and has a passion for fixing up houses and refinishing furniture. She also likes dog-walking, kayaking, skiing, Celtic dancing, singing and crafts.

She told her story from her home on the Pacific coast, listening to the waves lapping the shore.

Helen Sharpe

Helen is divorced, lives in Toronto, and has two sons and five grand-children. She was diagnosed in April 1973, a month before her 41st birthday. She describes herself before her diagnosis as a Jewish housewife who enjoyed perfect health and led a "full, well-rounded life as a wife, mother, volunteer, part-time university student and performer in amateur musical comedy." After her cancer experience Helen went back to school and obtained a degree in law. She is tall, slender and blond, and her children and friends describe her as "independent, funny, gutsy and outgoing." When Helen isn't working or dragon boating with Dragons Abreast, she enjoys reading ("I am a voracious reader"), traveling to Israel and spending time with family and friends.

Helen's storytelling place is a bower in a garden where cardinals land and the air is fragrant with the scent of lily of the valley and lilacs – flowers that bring her back to childhood places where she felt loved, peaceful and happy.

Brenda Tierney

Brenda is married and lives in Burnaby, B.C. Her son was 16 when she was diagnosed twelve years ago. She is blond, small-boned and medium height, "with stamina rather than strength!" Brenda loves to laugh and enjoy life. She gets her spiritual strength from the beauty of the world, and she is an avid hiker. Her friends are important to her and they tell her that she is a good listener, with a great sense of humor and keen perceptions. Brenda recently became the first treasurer of the Vancouver dragon boating society, Abreast in a Boat.

She told her story from the summit of a nearby mountain – "worth the exhausting hike because of the beauty that waits at the top."

Fran Weiss

Fran is married and lives in Winnipeg with "the kindest of husbands and an exciting 17-year-old daughter." She is the mother of six children between the ages of 17 and 37, and a registered nurse by profession. Fran was diagnosed in March 1997 just as she was turning 60. In the aftermath of her cancer experience she joined the Winnipeg team Chemo Savvy. Her friends identify Fran as "optimistic and positive, always able to find the glass half full." She describes herself as "wiry and energetic" – her uncle nicknamed her "Frantic Franny" when she was a child. She is a good organizer and leader, loves music, and serves as an organist, choir singer and music director at her church. She enjoys cottage and city life, cross-country skiing, swimming, and especially hosting family and friends at home and at the lake.

She imagined telling her story from a bug-proof gazebo in her garden, surrounded by flowers and trees. As the listener gently asked the discerning questions, her story unfolded over many cups of herbal "philosopher's tea."

Brenda Welsh

Brenda lives in north Toronto with her husband, Stephen, and two "lazy" cats. She has 15 nieces and nephews and enjoys spending time with family and friends. Brenda has a master's degree in Social Work and works for the Children's Aid Society. She was 35 years old when she was diagnosed. Just prior to the diagnosis she was trying to conceive, but the chemotherapy treatment made her dream impossible. Brenda and Stephen are now in the process of adopting a little girl from China. She joined the Toronto team Dragons Abreast in 1998 and then began volunteering as a speaker for the Canadian Breast Cancer Foundation, Ontario Chapter. She says that her friends would probably describe her as "tenacious, hard-working, adventurous, kind and non-judgmental."

Her storytelling place was at the bottom of the sea, in the Great Barrier Reef, "brilliant in the reflected sunlight, with a myriad of colorful fish slowly dancing through the coral in all shapes and sizes. It was so quiet, calm and relaxing that I could actually hear the fish eating algae off the coral."

Pearls of Wisdom

What to Do if You Meet a Dragon

🌿 Meet it head on. Face it!

— *Pamela Robbins*

🌿 Introduce yourself as politely as you can.
Stand at a distance in case of fiery breath.
Tell him how handsome he is.

— *Marjorie Greenwood*

🌿 BE AFRAID. BE VERY AFRAID.

— *Marianne Primeau*

🌿 Stay calm and don't judge the fierceness of the dragon by
what it looks like.

— *Karen Kellner*

🌿 Remember, everything happens for a reason.

— *Helen Sharpe*

🌿 Ask him about himself.
Ask him not to breathe fire.

Ask for a free ride.
Invite him in for tea.
(Is there a *Mrs.* Dragon?)

– Fran Weiss

🌿 Pat the dragon on the head. According to legend, that is supposed to bring you luck. To ignore this ancient legend is to tempt fate!

– Evelyn Crofts

🌿 If you are attacked, don't wait too long before you have that wound checked out by your doctor.

– Chantal Brunet

🌿 Let it know who's boss. Always make direct eye contact.

– Cathy Prusak

🌿 Take a deep breath, stand back, and then start kicking!

– Brenda Welsh

🌿 Keep your wits about you.
Speak to it calmly and gently.
Examine the dragon in detail, notice every wart and mole.

– Akky Mansikka

🌿 Dare to smell his breath! If it's full of garlic, you will *know* he's on your side!

– Anita Ewart

🌿 Ask it if it will take you for a ride. (But don't aggravate it.)

– Brenda Tierney

What Not to Do if You Meet a Dragon

🍂 Don't run away or it will chase you.

— *Pamela Robbins*

🍂 Don't be rude.
Don't make nasty comments about his breath.
Don't ask what he thinks of St. George.

— *Marjorie Greenwood*

🍂 Do not smile.
Do not show any signs of weakness.
Do not look into its eyes!
And for heaven's sake, never feed it!

— *Marianne Primeau*

🍂 Never ignore something that looks like it might be a dragon.
Dragons most often come quietly and stealthily. They take
years to establish their lairs without our knowledge and then
suddenly burst forth, wreaking havoc in our lives and bodies.
Your best chance to beat the dragon is when it is young and
small.

— *Marian Busch*

🍂 Don't be afraid – he looks scarier than he is.

— *Helen Sharpe*

🍂 Don't be intimidated.
Don't run and hide.

— *Fran Weiss*

🍃 Never ignore a dragon if you are lucky enough to meet one, because that will only anger it. There's nothing nastier than an angry dragon. You'll end up in troubled waters for sure.

– Evelyn Crofts

🍃 Don't turn your back on a dragon. They can be very sneaky and may try to trip you.

– Cathy Prusak

🍃 Don't close your eyes and appear dead – he might eat you. Don't give up before the fight is over.

– Brenda Welsh

🍃 Never underestimate the power of a dragon.

– Barb Chomski

🍃 Don't scream and yell and stamp your feet. That is futile and will aggravate the beast.
Don't try to hide – the dragon knows where you are at all times.

– Akky Mansikka

🍃 Don't turn your back, as he'll likely either "fire you up" in ways you may *not* appreciate or he'll kick you so hard you won't be able to sit down to paddle and you'll miss the ride!

– Anita Ewart

How to Approach a Dragon

🍃 Approach slowly, at your own speed.

– Pamela Robbins

✺ Approach from behind, with caution. Stand tall.

– Marianne Primeau

✺ Be bold. Be relentless. Be confident. Remember that it's not over until you say it's over.

– Marian Busch

✺ Approach carefully, one breast at a time.

– Fran Weiss

✺ Show the dragon respect. Give it your focus. Remain silent, and speak when the dragon is ready to listen. When the time comes, you will know it.

– Evelyn Crofts

✺ Approach with respect. And be armed, just in case! Feel the area, make sure it is safe. Be positive and self-confident. If you show fear or are weak, the dragon will attack.

– Chantal Brunet

✺ Don't get too close, they tend to have bad breath.

– Cathy Prusak

✺ Approach with your eyes wide open.
Put on your armor and be prepared to fight.
Read as many books as possible on how to slay a dragon.
Welcome as many villagers as possible to help you with your quest.

– Brenda Welsh

✺ Approach the dragon with caution and respect, and keep out of range of his fire.

– Barb Chomski

🍂 Arm yourself with the facts. There are a lot of myths out there, and some can be harmful.
Some weapons are very effective, but some aren't. You have to face the dragon all by yourself, but it is comforting to know there are warriors that will back you up.

– Akky Mansikka

🍂 Ask questions, be wary, don't assume anything, and be ready for some changes in your life you may never have dreamed possible…

– Anita Ewart

🍂 Approach a dragon with courage and humor.

– Helen Sharpe

🍂 Approach a dragon gently and with consideration. After all, he is a revered animal in Chinese folklore and deserves courtesy.

– Kaethe Lawn

How to Tame a Dragon

🍂 Embrace it. Trust it.

– Pamela Robbins

🍂 Make friends with him. Ask him to protect you from harm.

– Marjorie Greenwood

🍂 Try hard to get to know the dragon, what it thinks, likes, dislikes, wants, and do this without upsetting the dragon.

– Marianne Primeau

❧ Ask it about itself. Ask it how it got its scales and wounds. Tell the dragon about your own scales and wounds. (When in doubt, hit him with a prosthesis!)

– Fran Weiss

❧ Be patient.
Give your heart to a dragon and you will most certainly tame the dragon. Once the dragon has your heart, he becomes a warrior and will champion any cause for you.

– Evelyn Crofts

❧ Show the dragon that you will not give up, that you will not surrender. When he attacks, attack back. Destroy any poison he has contaminated you with. Show him that you are a winner.

– Chantal Brunet

❧ Be firm and consistent. Don't rush things. Dragons can be quite stupid and they may take time to learn new concepts. The broncobusting technique may be worth a try; just get on and ride.

– Cathy Prusak

❧ Tame a dragon with knowledge, inner peace and a team of dragon warriors.

– Brenda Welsh

❧ I think I'd run up its tail if I had a chance, but it's probably pretty hard to sneak up on a dragon. Tame a dragon by making friends with it. This is risky, of course. I understand some dragons are quite cantankerous, and how would you really know if you had a happy one or a nasty one?

– Brenda Tierney

🍃 Make friends with your dragon and be gentle. Find out what his weakness is and be compassionate and understanding.

– *Barb Chomski*

🍃 Bring flowers and think of beautiful things. Beautiful things distract it and suck up some of its strength. Listen to music. Laughter totally confuses it and dilutes its power.

Once you get close, embrace the dragon. Tickle its tummy, make it laugh, for it can be humorous. Soothe it, hug it and love every aspect of it. Listen to it and learn to recognize its songs. You may not be able to hear them at first, but they will become louder and clearer.

If it gets out of control, find someone who will help you calm it down, and calm you down as well. Get used to how it feels, and let it feel you on its back. Get on slowly and feel it out. You'll be surprised how good it feels.

– *Akky Mansikka*

🍃 Recognize this new ally, respect him, get into the water with him often, laugh easily and frequently. Qu Yuan will hear you and rejoice!

– *Anita Ewart*

🍃 Tame him with your indomitable spirit.

– *Helen Sharpe*

How to Stay On for the Ride

𝕀 Become one with the dragon. You are not a separate entity. You are one entity. You are the heart of the dragon. To think of yourself as a separate entity is, once again, to tempt fate.

– *Evelyn Crofts*

𝕀 Have just enough self-confidence. Never forget that the dragon is a dragon and can turn around and be mean again. Keep your mind focused on each movement of the dragon. Keep your mind and your body in great shape in case you must fight again. Finally, hope for a dragon cure: one day, there will be a candy man giving out "goodies" (medication) to get rid of dragon poison and make sure it never affects you again. On that day life will never be the same ever after for all the women of the world!

– *Chantal Brunet*

𝕀 Buckle up. Wear a crash helmet in case of falls. Hang on tight!

– *Cathy Prusak*

𝕀 Don't kick it to make it go faster. They breathe fire. The only way you can stay on any animal is to grab the horns or ears or whatever is handy and wrap your legs around its neck and hold on.

– *Brenda Tierney*

𝕀 Hang on tight and enjoy the view. Go with the flow.

– *Barb Chomski*

🌿 Hold on tight, because you won't be used to how it moves. It is not as wild and erratic as you might think; there is a rhythm and predictability to the way it moves and sings.

Get right back on if you fall off. The dragon isn't going anywhere.

Be prepared to be taken to new worlds full of excitement and adventure. These new places and people may frighten you at first, but give them a chance. You are in for the ride of your life!

Get used to change, because once you get on, everything will constantly change. The dragon will change how you feel and see things, and that's all right. Hang on!

Laughter and fun keep the dragon on track and tame.

– Akky Mansikka

🌿 Keep yourself in good shape, exercise, eat and sleep well. Like yourself (because of, not in spite of, your altered shape) and love the world as much as you can.

Remember, today is a gift, *not* a given, so make the most of every day.

– Anita Ewart

🌿 Get on with your life, make plans, enjoy family and friends.

– Helen Sharpe

🌿 Get on and experience everything life has to offer. Ride him hard, work with him, love the sheer joy that the dragon will give you.

– Irene Hogendoorn

❦ Consider it a great honor to ride on his scaly back – even if you get wet!

Tell him that should he be willing to become your companion animal, you would feel most honored and would give him the utmost best of care.

– Kaethe Lawn

❦ Don't sweat the small stuff. Stay positive. You will find hope in unexpected places, so keep your eyes, ears and mind open.

– Marian Busch

❦ There is no crying in dragon boat racing, only tears of joy. It's not whether you win or lose, but to say, "Hey! I'm here and I'm *in* the race!"

– Marianne Primeau

❦ Take a fairly large foam cushion, those spikes can *smart!*

– Marjorie Greenwood

❦ Hang on tight. Go with the flow. Have faith, hope. The ride is bumpy, like a rollercoaster. But you adjust, learn to roll with it.

– Pamela Robbins

❦ Even when you feel backed up against a door, find a window.

– Brenda Welsh

Bibliography

Allen, Judy, and Griffiths, Jean. *The Book of the Dragon*. Secaucus, New Jersey: Chartwell Books, 1979.

Barker, Pat. *Dragon Boats: A Celebration*. Vancouver, B.C.: Raincoast Books, 1996.

Christie, Anthony. *Chinese Mythology*. London: The Hamlyn Publishing Group, 1975.

Cirlot, J.E. *A Dictionary of Symbols*. London: Routledge & Kegan Paul, 1962.

Crossley-Holland, Kevin, trans. *Beowulf: A Verse Translation*. New York: Oxford University Press, 1999.

Eliade, Mircea. *Myths, Dreams and Mysteries*. New York: Harper & Row, 1975.

Grimm, Jakob and Wilhelm. *The Complete Grimm's Fairy Tales*. New York: Pantheon Books, 1972.

Hays, Edward. *St. George and the Dragon and the Quest for the Holy Grail*. Leavenworth, Kansas: Forest of Peace Publishing, 1986.

Heaney, Seamus, trans. *Beowulf: A New Verse Translation*. New York: W. W. Norton & Company, 2000.

Ingersoll, Ernest. *Dragons and Dragon Lore*. Escondido, California: The Book Tree, 1999.

Jones, David E. *An Instinct for Dragons*. New York: Routledge, 2000.

Larsen, Stephen. *The Mythic Imagination, The Quest for Meaning through Personal Mythology*. Rochester, Vermont: Inner Traditions International, 1996

Love, Dr. Susan. *Dr. Susan Love's Breast Book*. Cambridge, Massachusetts: Perseus Publishing, 2000.

May, Rollo. *Freedom and Destiny*. New York: W.W. Norton & Company, 1999.

McKenzie, Dr. Donald C. "Abreast in a Boat – a race against breast cancer." *Canadian Medical Association Journal* (August 1988).

Newman, Paul. *The Hill of the Dragon: An Enquiry into the Nature of Dragon Legends*. Bath, U.K.: Kingsmead Press, 1979.

Nuland, Dr. Sherwin B. *How We Die: Reflections on Life's Final Chapter*. New York: Vintage Books, 1993.

Okakura, Kakasu. *The Awakening of Japan*. New York: Century Co., 1904.

Rebsamen, Frederick, trans. *Beowulf: A Verse Translation*. New York: HarperCollins Publishers, 1991.

Rilke, Rainer Maria. (John Mood, trans.) *Rilke on Love and Other Difficulties*. New York: W.W. Norton & Company, 1975.

Schucman, Helen, and Thetford, William. *A Course in Miracles*. Mill Valley, California: Foundation for Inner Peace, 1975.

Yang, Hsien-Yi, and Yang, Gladys, trans. *The Dragon King's Daughter: Ten Tang Dynasty Stories*. Beijing: Foreign Languages Press, 1980.